Overcoming Common Proble

D0718352

Overcoming Common Problems Series

How to Stick to a Diet
Deborah Steinberg and Dr Windy Dryden

How to Stop Worrying
Dr Frank Tallis

The How to Study Book
Alan Brown

How to Succeed as a Single Parent
Carole Baldock

How to Untangle Your Emotional Knots
Dr Windy Dryden and Jack Gordon

How to Write a Successful CV
Joanna Gutmann

Hysterectomy
Suzie Hayman

The Irritable Bowel Diet Book
Rosemary Nicol

The Irritable Bowel Stress Book
Rosemary Nicol

Is HRT Right for You?
Dr Anne MacGregor

Jealousy
Dr Paul Hauck

Living with Asthma
Dr Robert Youngson

Living with Crohn's Disease
Dr Joan Gomez

Living with Diabetes
Dr Joan Gomez

Living with Fibromyalgia
Christine Craggs-Hinton

Living with Grief
Dr Tony Lake

Living with High Blood Pressure
Dr Tom Smith

Living with Nut Allergies
Karen Evennett

Living with Osteoporosis
Dr Joan Gomez

Living with a Stoma
Dr Craig White

Making Friends with Your Stepchildren
Rosemary Wells

Motor Neurone Disease – A Family Affair
Dr David Oliver

Overcoming Anger
Dr Windy Dryden

Overcoming Anxiety
Dr Windy Dryden

Overcoming Guilt
Dr Windy Dryden

Overcoming Jealousy
Dr Windy Dryden

Overcoming Procrastination
Dr Windy Dryden

Overcoming Shame
Dr Windy Dryden

Overcoming Your Addictions
Dr Windy Dryden and
Dr Walter Matweychuk

The Parkinson's Disease Handbook
Dr Richard Godwin-Austen

The PMS Diet Book
Karen Evennett

A Positive Thought for Every Day
Dr Windy Dryden

Rheumatoid Arthritis
Mary-Claire Mason and Dr Elaine Smith

Second Time Around
Anne Lovell

Serious Mental Illness – A Family Affair
Gwen Howe

Shift Your Thinking, Change Your Life
Mo Shapiro

The Stress Workbook
Joanna Gutmann

The Subfertility Handbook
Virginia Ironside and Sarah Biggs

Successful Au Pairs
Hilli Matthews

Talking with Confidence
Don Gabor

Ten Steps to Positive Living
Dr Windy Dryden

Think Your Way to Happiness
Dr Windy Dryden and Jack Gordon

The Travellers' Good Health Guide
Ted Lankester

Understanding Obsessions and Compulsions
Dr Frank Tallis

Understanding Sex and Relationships
Rosemary Stones

Understanding Your Personality
Patricia Hedges

Work–Life Balance
Gordon and Ronni Lamont

Overcoming Common Problems

Hysterectomy

What it is and how to cope with it successfully

Suzie Hayman

6/505955

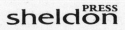

sheldon **PRESS**

First published in Great Britain in 1986 by
Sheldon Press
Holy Trinity Church
Marylebone Road
London NW1 4DU

Revised 1994

New edition 2002

British Library Cataloguing-in-Publication Data

A catalogue record for this book is available from the British Library

ISBN 0–85969–870–X

Typeset by Deltatype Limited, Birkenhead, Merseyside
Printed in Great Britain by Biddles Ltd
www.biddles.co.uk

Contents

Acknowledgements

I would like to thank the people who helped make sure my hysterectomy left no scars, either physical or emotional:

Robin Ballard, a gynaecologist *par excellence*, who earned trust and affection by offering respect and a listening ear.

Vic Cowan, the best of all men, who was loving, caring and encouraging.

The staff and my fellow patients at St Mary's, Roehampton, who were always ready with sympathy and understanding.

Introduction

Every week, over 1500 women in the United Kingdom have a hysterectomy – an operation to remove their uterus or womb. Hysterectomy is the fifth most common operation in this country. Currently, every woman has a one in five chance of having a hysterectomy at some time in her life. In fact, it's estimated that today's teenage girl will have a one in eight chance of losing her womb by the time she is 50.

In most cases, surgery isn't because of a life-threatening condition. It's usually recommended or decided upon by the woman's doctor because she is suffering from something that makes her life difficult or miserable. In some cases, it is because she has made the *doctor's* life miserable. She may have made frequent visits, presenting symptoms for which he has no explanation or cure. If these centre around period pain or heavy bleeding, a hysterectomy may seem the best solution. When weighing up the choices, most doctors only consider the physical aspect. On the face of it, a hysterectomy is just like removing the appendix or tonsils. It's an operation to take away an organ which is causing problems, and losing that organ doesn't affect the body in any way. But a woman's womb means far, far more to her than her tonsils or her appendix. Too few of us have the self-confidence to insist that our emotions *are* a factor. Possession of a womb – even one that refuses to function properly – is an important part of our self-image.

This book aims to introduce you to your womb, to explain how it functions and what can go wrong with it. We shall explore how a doctor would diagnose problems with the womb and how they may be treated, with and without surgery. We shall see how you would prepare for a hysterectomy, and exactly what would happen while you were in hospital and after your release. The fears you and your partner might have about the operation itself and the long-term consequences will be discussed. You'll have the facts. You'll also have the reassuring knowledge that all these 'irrational' worries are shared by all women and their families, and are quite legitimate. You should be able to ask for a say in whether or not you have a hysterectomy, and be able to cope if it does happen to you.

1

More Than Just a Surgical Procedure

By the time I saw the hospital doctor, I knew that there was something seriously wrong and that my womb would have to go. I can't describe the feelings of horror, of desolation almost, that hit me when he said, 'It'll have to come out, Mrs B.' What was so awful was that he quite obviously thought I was being silly to feel upset. I'd had my family, it was a useless and even dangerous part – why not whip it out? I just couldn't explain that it was *me*, the centre of my whole life, that he was wanting to slice out and throw away.

Sally B

The feelings a woman has for her womb are quite unlike the relationship she has with any other part of her body. The human body is a masterpiece of engineering, with impressive 'back-up' systems. You could lose part of a kidney, sections of lung, yards of gut, even portions of brain tissue, and still survive quite well, with few physical or emotional ill-effects. There is even one organ – the appendix – you don't use at all. The appendix was necessary when our ancestor was a grass-eating animal. The appendix helped to digest the cellulose in grass. Now, the appendix is no longer needed and can be removed with no effect on the workings of the body. When faced with a woman whose family is complete and whose womb is giving problems, many doctors will treat this organ as if it were an appendix. They feel it is a useless, redundant bit of your body you no longer need or want.

Unfortunately, few women see their womb in this light. From the day your periods start, you may have developed a complex love/hate relationship with your womb. It gives you cramping pains and a monthly flow that can be smelly, uncomfortable and embarrassing. But this monthly blood is also a symbol. Starting your periods shows you've become an adult. For some, the monthly cycle is a burden. Periods make you feel dirty and give

1

you headaches, mood changes and discomfort. Others, however, find they feel extra sexy and 'high' during their periods or midway between them. You may see your periods as the 'curse', or just a fact of life. What you can't escape from is the fact that, from your teenage years on, for a quarter of your life your womb will remind you each month that it's there.

We might have grumbled about periods when we were teenagers. The chances are we would have been told, 'Never mind, it shows you are a woman, you can have babies.' Puberty brings periods and the ability to become pregnant. It also brings up the subject of sex. These elements all combine, and we see them as being connected. Being feminine means being able to bear children → means having monthly periods → means being feminine. To many of us, these ideas are like a house of cards. We think, 'Remove one, and the others come tumbling down.' 'Proper' women, 'real' women, have babies, or at least the potential to do so. If you can't get pregnant you, and other people, may feel you are not sexually complete, not satisfactorily feminine. Even if you have already *had* children, taking away your womb feels like taking away your womanliness.

Women are usually perfectly happy to get rid of periods. It is what our periods signify that is difficult to part with. If, deep down, you see being a mother and wife as the most important part of your self, losing your womb feels like losing part of your identity. Many of us believe the most fulfilling job for a woman is to be a mother. Some people still think it's the only one women should do! If motherhood is an important part of the way you see yourself, a hysterectomy is a real loss. It takes away and destroys your qualifications and your work tools. Your womb is your reason for being who you are and where you are. You may have had no intention of putting it to work again. Even so, the fact that it was there ready to be called upon gave you 'job security' and a right to the status of mother/woman/wife. Because of this, there are scores of myths about the effects and meaning of a hysterectomy. Having had one, say the mythmakers, 'You can never be the same again', 'You're no good because you can never have children again', 'You're less of a woman', 'Sex is over for

2

you' and 'You'll become masculine'. *None of these is true!* But
many people believe them. This shows how very insecure we can
feel about problems that affect our ability to enjoy sex or have
children.

Some men seem to find it difficult to understand these fears.
Which is strange, since they suffer from exactly the same worries.
Men whose wives don't get pregnant are often laughed at by
friends for not being able to 'get it up'. Their shame and fear
often *can* lead to sexual difficulties. Yet a man can be totally
sterile and not even know it. He can still go on having erections
and enjoying lovemaking. Even having a testicle removed need
make no difference to his sexual performance or his fertility. Men
can have all sorts of fears about their ability to make love and get
their partners pregnant. So you'd think most of them would
understand and be sympathetic to a woman's worries about sex
and pregnancy. However, when a man feels unable or unwilling
to have sex, you can see it. He won't be able to perform. Even
when she doesn't fancy it, a woman can still go through the
motions. Perhaps this is why the average man finds it difficult to
take women's fears as seriously as his own. Or maybe the reason
men often don't seem to think about these subjects is that it's just
too scary.

Doctors can shy off thinking or talking about your emotional
reactions, too. Some don't seem to realize how you will feel
when they tell you that you need a hysterectomy. Most would
accept that it's a medical and a personal tragedy for a young
woman to have to lose her womb before she has had her children.
But they may think that if you are in your forties or older, with
several children, it doesn't matter so much. You may well find a
gynaecologist treats a hysterectomy as no more than a routine
medical procedure. This can lead to a situation where doctor and
patient misunderstand each other. They may act as if they know it
all, but doctors are human, too. *Any* situation where a doctor tells
a patient that he or she is ill and needs surgery is charged with
emotion. Doctors try to remain distant and objective. They want
to keep control and make the best decisions possible for their
patient. So they don't want to become emotionally involved in

3

any way. But hysterectomy is even more emotional than most operations. Most of us get worried about anything to do with sex, and doctors may do, too. They often deal with this by stepping backwards. They avoid hearing, and understanding, the fears you have about the news that you have an illness and need major surgery. When you ask questions, they may slap a label on you. They could say you're being 'neurotic' and 'female' and 'emotional', rather than sensible and normal to be concerned. You may find that the more you ask questions or show concern, the more a doctor becomes set on doing a hysterectomy – as if removing your womb won't only remove your symptoms, but also all your fears and problems. Which could be fine, except your fears aren't 'symptoms' but a reasonable reaction to the idea of having surgery. Your 'cure' would be a full explanation of why the operation is necessary, how it will affect you and what alternatives there may be.

On the other hand, some women find that expressing doubts and asking questions gets them refused an operation they might need. You may be marked down in hospital notes as being unable to come to terms with the operation. Some doctors still find it difficult to accept women as mature, thinking beings. They may insist that, once having had doubts, you rule yourself out. If you protest that, having had a chance to discuss and think it over, you would now like the operation, they may not listen. You're only an emotional woman, and he knows best!

There is no doubt that hysterectomy is not always the answer to menstrual problems. Periods can become heavy and painful for emotional as well as physical reasons. Removing the womb in such a case only removes the symptoms, leaving the problem intact. Pre-menstrual tension can continue, even when the womb has been taken out. However, for some women, their depression and stress is a result of period problems, not the cause. To be told, 'Taking your womb away will not cure your depression. Let's wait until you are better,' is insulting and doesn't help.

Reactions to hysterectomy

Many women feel ignored and patronized by doctors. They feel some doctors take their fears and feelings lightly. The problem is that the attitudes of your doctors, friends and family are very important. They can have as much an effect on the outcome of your operation as the surgeon's technical skills. There are studies that suggest that as many as 70 per cent of hysterectomy patients suffer depression. But other studies come up with far lower figures. Hysterectomy *need* be no more traumatic than any other operation. How you react to your hysterectomy will probably depend on four elements.

The amount of information you are given
Women whose questions about the operation and its effects are answered have far fewer problems afterwards than women kept in ignorance. The same is true about women who know how their own bodies work. You owe it to yourself to persist. If you are unlucky enough to have doctors and nurses who seem to believe that it is *their* job to look after you and *your* job to be quiet and looked after, keep asking! It is *your* body that is being worked on. You have every right to be an equal partner in every step from diagnosis to cure.

The amount of support you have from family and friends
It goes without saying that you have a better chance of recovery if you do not have to rise early from a sickbed to cook, clean and generally look after other people. But *emotional* support is even more important. It is bad enough that *you* feel that something vital has been removed from you. You'll find it far easier to regain your physical and emotional health if your friends and, most important, your sexual partner, are supportive and positive.

The reason for your operation
Losing your womb is a blow. But you'll feel far better about it if your doctors can tell you they found physical proof that it was essential. Women who have had hysterectomies for vague

5

reasons often feel cheated. If yours was for heavy or irregular periods for which the doctors could find no obvious cause you may find it harder to accept. It is a horrible thought that you might have gone through all this for nothing. However worried or unhappy you might feel about a hysterectomy, if you felt you had no choice you may feel reassured. Then, you know that hysterectomy was the best or the only option. Your womb is a fair price to pay for your health or even your life.

Your general state of mind and situation in life

There are certain things that may make it more likely that one woman finds it harder to cope than another. If you're a worrier, a hysterectomy may leave you feeling on edge and concerned. If you have areas of unhappiness in your life – doubts about yourself or your marriage – a hysterectomy will not cure them. Some women put all their energy and self-image into being a mother, and pay less attention to their own lives and needs. They may feel a strong sense of loss. If your religion teaches you that sex is mainly for the creation of life, or you still do want another child, you may find sexual activity after the operation makes you feel guilty or empty.

Some of these four elements are beyond your control. But most of them are not. When you understand *why* you and others react in a certain way, you can often think your way through it. You may not be able to throw off the results of years of belief, but you can, perhaps, come to terms with it. On the practical side, you see why it is so important for you to find out as much as possible about your body, your illness and your operation. And for you to talk openly to people whose behaviour and attitudes will have an important effect on your future health.

2
Your Partner's Fears

I don't really know how he feels about the operation. When I told him the doctor said I had to have it, he just shrugged. We haven't really talked about it at all.

Anne T

I suppose I just found the whole thing embarrassing. We don't really talk about these things. We've only made love a few times since she came out of hospital and I know she thinks I've gone off her. I haven't, well not really. I can't explain how I feel – don't know myself.

Anthony T

It may seem fairly obvious that your operation is going to affect people other than you. If you have a family, their daily routines will be upset while you're in hospital and as you recover at home afterwards. Friends and colleagues at work will have to make allowances for you. But the practical details aren't the only aspect to think about. It can be easy to miss the fact that your hysterectomy will mean a lot more than having to change their habits for a few weeks. Any operation, and especially one that leaves you so noticeably weak, can be terrifying to children. Young people fancy that the most important people in the world – themselves, their parents and grandparents – will never really fall seriously ill or die. A hysterectomy and its after-effects can scarily suggest they can. When something strikes at your deepest fears, it is a very common reaction to close your eyes and pretend it's not really there. So your family may act as if nothing is wrong, which can hurt and confuse you. Your kids may act bored when they visit you in hospital. They may even insist on leaving early so as not to miss a favourite television programme. As soon as you get home, they may be amazed and furious if everything is not back to normal at once. Don't take it personally. You don't have a house full of unfeeling monsters. What's hidden behind this 'selfishness' is an overwhelming fear. They're terrified that maybe you *will* die and leave them. Maybe it *was* their fault, for working you too hard. Maybe, if they carry on as normal, this will prove they are not to blame and the whole nasty nightmare will disappear.

Your partner's fears

At the centre of all this can be your sexual partner. The greatest fear of most women having a hysterectomy is that the operation will destroy their femininity and sexual appeal. This is true whether they are straight or gay. Your sexual identity – whether you see yourself as someone who is, and should be, able to give and receive sexual pleasure – is often a result of your upbringing and adult sexual experiences. You can be warm and sensuous and happy to see yourself as a sexy person, even if your parents and any partners thought sex was dirty and something not to be talked about! But few of us are so confident and comfortable in our sexuality that the attitudes of those we love have no effect. You could bounce out of hospital convinced that a hysterectomy has left your essential womanliness untouched. But if your partner's first reaction is to draw back in revulsion or say, 'You're less of a woman now,' you'd feel down. Your partner's beliefs will have an enormous influence on your self-esteem after the operation. And so too will the beliefs of friends, colleagues and relatives. You will need to understand that men, too, have fears about hysterectomy. They are quite likely to have confused ideas about why yours was necessary. If your partner is male, he may be wondering what part he had to play in your illness and how it might now harm him.

Hysterectomy and sexuality

The perils of sex are the one form of sex education most of us have received. Sex, we are told, can give you sexual infections and cancer. It does not take much to turn this round and give you the nagging fear that *any* disorder of your sex parts must therefore be due to sex. If you are gay, you may be feeling that the condition that led to a hysterectomy might be a punishment or result of your sexuality. If you are straight, you may lean towards the view that sex is something a man does and a woman accepts, rather than an experience both enjoy with equal satisfaction. If you think about it this way you could feel that if he's 'inflicted' sex, then he's also 'caused' the illness. Either his over-enthusiastic behaviour has torn her inside, or his body fluids have given her cancer or some other disease. Whether your sex life is still an active one or your relationship has become loving and companionable, these fears can influence what happens after a hysterectomy.

Men are brought up on a diet of myths about their sexuality. Many of the words and phrases they learn as children and teenagers to describe their equipment and activity sound violent and powerful. A boy is said to 'have the horn' or be 'horny', have a 'hard on' or even a 'dagger', if he is sexually excited. His penis is a 'cock' or a 'prick'. Sex is called 'having a woman' or 'having it off' or even 'ploughing her'. A woman may bleed the first time she has sex. With this and the background of these sharp, attacking words, it is hardly surprising that some men are convinced that their sexual urges have the strength to inflict great damage on their partners. If many women have only a vague idea of how their bodies work and what exactly is inside them, men are even more in the dark. The news that their partner has 'something wrong in there' and that these parts are so damaged that they have to be removed can give rise to terrible feelings of guilt. The man who complains about how his wife's stay in hospital will inconvenience him may not be unfeeling and selfish. He may be trying to say, 'This is all my fault, but I can't bear to think about it. Perhaps if I can make *you* feel guilty about leaving me alone, we can both forget the fact that I'm the one who is really to blame.'

It is very common for men who have been unable to discuss their feelings about their wives' hysterectomies to have emotional difficulties after the event. When his partner returns from hospital with the news that sex is banned for at least six weeks, these fears are confirmed. If his sexual advances can damage her now, this

9

proves that it was his sexual behaviour that probably caused the problem in the first place! Depression, attempts at suicide and bouts of anger have all been reported. Some men are unable to perform sexually when their wives are given the all-clear by the hospital. They are so convinced that their erect penis will harm the person they love, or they are so overcome with guilt, that they become impotent. Others have promiscuous affairs. It is as if they are saying, 'It's not my fault – look at all these women I can have sex with, without them coming to harm.'

If you and your partner already have areas of conflict, you might find yourself encouraging these unspoken fears. If sex has never been particularly joyful, or has become unexciting in the last few years, this could be the perfect excuse to put it behind you. If you have felt that your partner has always taken advantage of you, the realization that he feels uncomfortable about your illness may tempt you to turn the tables.

Your partner could also have fears about his own wellbeing. When it comes to illness, many of us go back to our most primitive beliefs. Being in the same room or touching someone with cancer can fill us with terror, even though we *know* the disease is not catching. Having sexual intercourse is a far more intimate way of touching and one that puts your partner's most vulnerable parts at risk. If he believes that your operation has de-womanized you, he may fancy that such contact will un-man him. He may also be convinced that the removal of your womb will leave a gaping hole inside you. What, he may wonder, will happen to him if he does enter you? Will he be sucked in and lost inside? Instead of the firm grainy walls that used to grip his penis, will you be harsh like a scab or pulpy like an open wound? If you are now 'empty', will either of you get any satisfaction from making love?

Discussing the operation with your partner

Many hospitals and family doctors make the mistake of not fully involving your partner in the discussions about your illness. Partly, this is entirely reasonable. It is your body. You and your doctor are the only ones who should be involved in decisions about your health. But your family's attitudes will influence your recovery as much as your spell in hospital. Your partner shouldn't be able to interfere with your treatment, or override your wishes. But you would benefit if he were able to understand what is going on and both of you were able to express and share your impressions. There are, of course, practical difficulties. If he is working in clinic times, your partner is unlikely to be able to come with you on the visits to the hospital or to your own doctor. Nurses and doctors, who do not have to deal with the emotional results of hysterectomies, may not see counselling families and husbands as a priority in their very busy working lives. Some do make a point of calling in a husband and giving him a little talk about looking after the wife when she gets home. Very, very few acknowledge, or even understand, the confused fears these men will have. And very few men will be able to overcome their embarrassment and explain, especially when they themselves are probably unable to pinpoint exactly why the whole situation makes them feel uneasy. If you are in a same-sex relationship, it could on one level be easier. Another woman may be able to put herself in your shoes and understand your feelings better. But it may be even harder, in that some of the nurses and doctors you deal with could be unwilling to recognize that another woman is your partner and should be involved.

In most cases, it will be left to you to decide whether to discuss all this with your partner. You may come up against hostility or a blank wall. If your partner is a man, he may insist, 'I don't want to know about all that – it's women's business' or 'Spare me the awful details, that sort of thing just makes me ill.' You may need to ask your family doctor or district nurse or a good friend to help the two of you talk it out. However awkward and difficult it may be, helping him to understand your fears and letting him know you understand his can make an enormous difference. Some women find they can bring the subject up in conversation and their partners will discuss it. Others need to get the initial point across by writing a letter for their husbands to read in private, and then talk it over later on. Men who find the whole subject particularly stressful may still be willing to read books, magazine articles or leaflets. Although they cannot bring themselves to speak openly, they will take notice. Information about your body, your illness, your operation and both of your feelings about all these will allow him to appreciate your needs and his reactions. He will know why you need rest and help after the operation without having to feel this is a reflection on his earlier treatment of you. Both of you will be allowed to approach getting back to having sex with mutual understanding, tolerance and even humour. He will be transformed from a helpless onlooker to an essential support.

A hysterectomy is not a situation where 'Least said, soonest mended' is at all a helpful motto. The more you and your family can bring your ideas into the open and talk about them freely, the more chance you all have of recovering quickly and completely from this event.

3

Your Womb – What It Is and What It Does

> It took me two years to make my doctor listen to me and take me seriously. The main problem was that I really knew nothing about my own body, so when he said it was all in my mind, I didn't know enough to argue with him.
>
> *Betty S*

Hysterectomy, the name for the operation that removes a woman's womb or uterus, comes from the Greek for uterus – *hustera*. It used to be thought that a woman's womb controlled her mind and her emotions. Eighteenth-century doctors invented the word 'hysteria' to describe the state in which a woman appeared out of control or in great distress. To them, this *was* a mental disease caused by a disorder of the uterus. Even today, the word 'hysterical' is used to describe foolish female behaviour. Unfortunately, this earlier belief also led doctors to dismiss real and distressing symptoms as being 'hysterical' or 'all in the mind'. There are still some doctors who refuse to take their women patients seriously, saying that they are 'over-reacting' or being 'emotional' when they report pain or depression. These prejudices are helped by the fact that the functions and workings of the womb are largely controlled by hormonal changes. Hormones are chemical substances which trigger not only physical reactions in our bodies, but also emotional ones. Fortunately, more and more doctors are now recognizing that moodiness or depression can often be a symptom that should be taken seriously and not dismissed as a sign of foolishness, weakness or mental illness.

The uterus and its function

To understand what might go wrong with your womb or its related organs and so why you might need a hysterectomy, you first need to know how it acts in its normal state. Unlike most

13

vital organs, such as the heart, liver, kidneys or stomach, the womb is not necessary for your day-to-day survival. Strictly speaking, you could pass your whole life without using the womb for its one specific job, and not come to harm. The purpose of the uterus is to protect and nourish a baby. Each month, it prepares a home for a fertilized egg. The lining of your womb thickens and gets ready. Each month, if no egg arrives, this lining comes away as a period, and the process begins again. However, just because this function is not *essential* to your body, this does not mean that it has no impact. The monthly cycle has a powerful physical influence, both on your body and on your feelings. The possibility of pregnancy has a vital importance to every woman, as we have already discussed.

Where is the uterus found in the body, and what does it look like? It is about the size of your clenched fist, some 8 to 12 cm long and about 5 cm broad at the top. During pregnancy, it will stretch to contain the growing baby. After birth, it will shrink again but will remain a few centimetres longer than before you became pregnant. The uterus is shaped like a pear and lies in your pelvic cavity, midway between your hips. The 'stem' of this pear is the cervix or neck of the womb, which juts down into the vagina or sex passage. The cervix points downwards and backwards towards your buttocks, while the broad end of our imaginary pear slants forwards towards your navel or belly button. The uterus does not float in a hollow, but is cushioned on all sides. Below is the vagina, behind is the rectum or back passage, above are the coils of your bowel, and to the front is your bladder.

The uterus has three openings. At the stem end, the cervix provides a narrow channel down to the vagina. It is up through this that sperm may swim. At the top of the uterus, two openings extend on either side into the Fallopian tubes. It is down these that an egg will make its journey from the ovaries.

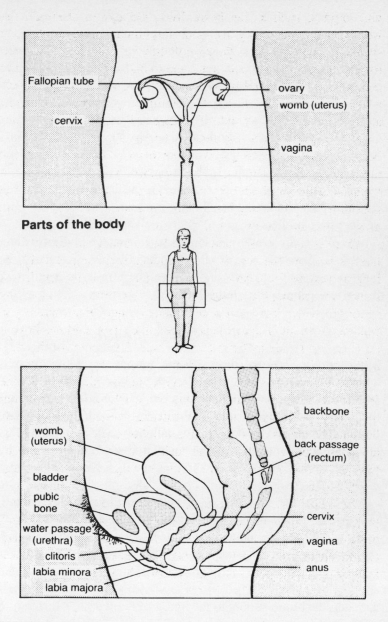

Parts of the body

The uterus is held in place by eight ligaments, which are bands of strong tissue. These stretch across the cavity from the bladder, the rectum and the walls of the pelvis. As well as holding the uterus in place, they secure the ovaries and Fallopian tubes. The ligaments keep the uterus in position, but not fixed rigidly. In fact, the uterus moves a great deal. It may be pushed by the surrounding organs, or move in response to the flexing of the elastic ligaments. Its position can also depend on how your body is standing or lying. When you lie on your back, your womb settles down towards your spine. When you stand, it drops a few centimetres. During sexual excitement, the ligaments tighten to lift the uterus so that the penis will have more room and not push against it. The state of the bladder or rectum will also have an effect. When the bladder is empty, the uterus will lie forward, across the flattened bag. As the bladder fills, the womb will be pushed gradually upwards and backwards. Similarly, a full back passage will push the uterus forwards.

How the uterus is formed

The uterus is made of blood, tissue, muscle, lymphatic vessels and nerves. These are formed in three layers. The first is a smooth, rubbery coat called peritoneum. Next is a layer of muscle interleaved with blood and lymphatic vessels and nerves. Unlike muscles in other parts of the body, such as legs or arms, these flex and contract in response to chemical messages rather than by your decision. Some of these muscles run as a band up the front of the uterus, over the top and down back to the cervix. They are extremely strong and can contract powerfully. During labour, they perform their most important job of squeezing rhythmically to force out the fully developed baby. They do a similar job each month, flexing to force out the cast-off lining of the womb as period blood. Scattered throughout the tissue of the uterus there are smaller muscles. Their job is to shut off small blood vessels and stop the blood supply to the lining of the womb, causing it to decay and come away each month. They also contract at the end of the period to stop further bleeding. The third layer making up

16

the uterus is mucous membrane. It is this that thickens every month to create the endometrium or lining of the womb.

The ovaries and hormones

Each month, a tiny gland at the base of the brain, called the pituitary, produces a chemical messenger or hormone. This is called *follicle stimulating hormone* or FSH. It is carried in your blood to your ovaries or egg cases. Each ovary contains thousands of immature or half-grown eggs. FSH triggers several tiny follicles or sacs to form on the surface of the almond-shaped ovaries, each sac bringing one egg to maturity. After a few days, the follicles send out their own hormone, oestrogen. The oestrogen does two things. First, it encourages the uterus to start growing a lining. Second, it tells the pituitary to stop sending FSH and instead produce another hormone – *luteinizing hormone* or LH; this new hormone acts on the follicles. Approximately 14 days after the pituitary first sent a message, one sac will burst and send a mature egg down one of the Fallopian tubes. This is *ovulation*.

The ovary now produces progesterone as well as oestrogen and the two hormones prepare the lining of the womb to become an inviting and nourishing home for a fertilized egg. If the egg meets acceptable sperm during the next 24 hours, conception will take place. The fertilized egg will drift down the tube, taking about seven days for its journey, and eventually be embedded in the womb wall. It will send out its own hormonal message, persuading the ovaries to continue sending the necessary hormones to keep the womb lining in place. If you do not become pregnant, the supplies of these hormones become less and, 14 days after ovulation, the womb lining will shed as blood and tiny clots of tissue – a 'period' or menstruation.

The shape and 'feel' of the uterus will change, during your monthly cycle and during your life. It becomes larger and rounder when you have a period. A doctor can detect a pregnancy even before the womb starts to grow noticeably bigger because the uterine muscles become firmer.

The menopause, and afterwards

Your reproductive organs do not 'wither away' when you go through the menopause. The menopause, when your periods stop, is only one aspect of the climacteric. The climacteric, which can take around five to ten years, usually occurs in your forties or fifties. The climacteric is part of a gradual slide from your having the potential to become pregnant to being no longer fertile. The menopause, when periods stop, occurs about midway through the process. During this time your ovaries will slowly stop sending out oestrogen and your hormonal system will adjust to this drop. The uterus and ovaries will shrink slightly and become paler in colour. More alarming and noticeable to the woman and her partner may be the fact that the vagina can also respond to a lack of oestrogen. The vaginal tissue can become dry and fragile, making sex painful. The delicate tissues of both vagina and urethra can be easily damaged, leading to infections. However, this need only be a temporary state of affairs. The female body survives perfectly well with these internal organs in 'retirement'. If you go on having regular sex, you'll find the vaginal tissue will stay comfortable and moist. If you stop having sex for a time, lubricating cream or gel can get you started again until the vagina gets moist on its own.

This, then, is the uterus and its related organs in its normal state. In the next chapter we will explore the many things that can go wrong and how these problems might make themselves felt.

4

Why You May Need a Hysterectomy – and Alternatives

I'd been having heavy periods for quite a few years. My GP sent me to hospital three years ago, but they weren't very helpful. Since then, I've been admitted twice as an emergency case because of heavy bleeding and I've had two D and Cs. The whole thing is really wearing me down. From one month to the next, I don't know whether I'll be flooding and exhausted for days, or OK. I've begged the consultant to do a hysterectomy, but he won't. He says, 'You're 51, it will sort itself out in time.' The problem is that I don't think I can stand the waiting!

Maureen W

The medical conditions which may make a doctor suggest a hysterectomy can be grouped under two loose categories. The first are identifiable conditions. The second are 'disorders'. Under identifiable conditions, one can put cancer, endometriosis, pelvic inflammatory disease, fibromyomata (fibroids) and prolapse of the womb. Under disorders, one can list difficulties with menstruation – painful, heavy or frequent bleeding. Some of the illnesses included under identifiable conditions *can* become dangerous and threaten a woman's life or her physical wellbeing. Those that come under the heading of disorders are less dangerous but more of a problem. The threat they pose is often more to her emotional wellbeing. They are often less easy to pinpoint by either patient or doctor. The attitudes of both women and their doctors play a part in whether help is requested, and the sort of help that is offered. Several Canadian, American and British studies have shown that which hospital or doctor a woman visits has as much influence on whether she has a hysterectomy or not as her medical condition. Some doctors appear to be 'hysterectomy-prone'. A leading doctor even dubbed one English

19

town 'Wombless Woking' for this reason. Some women are 'hysterectomy-prone', too. You might expect that women who have had one or more D and C or 'womb scrape' would be likely to end up having a hysterectomy. But it would appear that women making several visits in a year for vague symptoms are also likely to end up on the gynaecological surgery list. There are doctors who even say that you can predict whether a woman will eventually have this operation by measuring the thickness of her medical notes – the thicker they are, the more likely she is to be a hysterectomy patient in time.

Diagnosis

When a woman approaches her doctor, there are three levels of examination the doctor can do to decide whether there's a problem and what it is. The first is to consider what you have to tell about your problem. The doctor will 'take a history', or discuss with you your symptoms, past illnesses and sometimes the health of your immediate family. Menstrual problems, for instance, are often more likely to happen to you if your mother or sister suffered the same difficulties. You might be asked to give a specimen of your urine or water. Sometimes, the doctor asks for a *midstream urine* or MSU sample. This means they want a few drops of your water from halfway through emptying your bladder. You may be able to pass a few drops, stop and direct a few more drops into the bowl or bottle they give you, and finish into the lavatory. If once you start you keep on going, you should try to catch some of the stream after you have begun. At other times, they need *early morning* urine. This means the sample must be taken from the first time you go to the lavatory when you wake up in the morning.

Next, the doctor will want to do an internal examination. Many women are unhappy about these examinations. You might feel embarrassed at the intimacy involved in allowing a doctor to see what most of us consider 'private' parts of our body. You may also fear that the procedure will be painful. Both fears are understandable. However, a doctor is trained to look at you objectively, to see your body as a medical puzzle he or she must solve. They won't be making personal judgements or looking at you sexually. Looking up your vagina is no more 'intimate' to a doctor than looking up your nose. Vaginal examinations can be uncomfortable, but you can help to make them painless. The trick is not to tense up your muscles. To loosen yourself up, try taking several deep breaths and then let yourself go 'floppy' as you breathe out. Reminding yourself, 'This will only take a few minutes and is doing me good,' can also help.

The doctor will probably start by putting an instrument called a *speculum* into your vagina. A speculum is made of metal or plastic and looks like two spoons or scoops with long-handled bowls hinged together. The doctor slides the spoon end into the flexible tube that is your vagina. The doctor can then separate the speculum at the hinge, push the walls gently aside and see right up to the end of your vagina. The doctor can see the cervix where it juts into the vagina, and the tiny channel or 'os' which leads into the uterus. He or she can see whether there are any signs of damage or disease. The doctor can pass a smooth wooden stick up your vagina and, by gently rubbing this across the cervix, collect dead cells. This is the *Pap* (Papanicolaou) or *smear* test. The cells are treated and then sent off to be examined under a microscope. Minute changes will show whether they are normal, cancerous or becoming so (precancerous).

Having examined the sides of the vagina to make sure they are a healthy colour, the doctor will probably remove the speculum and do a bi-manual or two-handed examination. The doctor inserts one or two fingers into your vagina and puts the flats of the fingers of the other hand on your abdomen or tummy. By pressing the two hands together, the doctor can feel your uterus, Fallopian tubes, ovaries and other organs under the layers of skin and muscle. If you can imagine what it is like trying to find your keys, pencil and purse in a large bag, while wearing gloves and being blindfold, you will understand why a doctor needs experience and training to understand your body! If there are any lumps or swellings, or if the uterus is unexpectedly hard, this would alert the doctor to a problem. In some situations, the doctor may even have to put a finger up your rectum or back passage. This is because the vagina is about 10 cm long. If the doctor needs to feel further into your body than can be reached through the vagina the best way to do so is up the back passage.

Internal examinations

ratchet

bills

Speculum

Bi-manual examination

Vaginal examination, using a speculum

If, at the end of this examination, your doctor needs more information, you may be sent to see a specialist or gynaecologist in hospital. The gynaecologist will probably repeat the process and might also send you for an *ultrasound scan*. In this, sound waves are passed through your body and these build up a picture of your internal organs on a screen. A skilful operator can spot any unusual lumps or patches in your pelvis from this picture. You may also be asked to come in overnight for some checks under anaesthesia. While you are unconscious, the surgeon may pass a thin instrument up your vagina, through the narrow passage – the 'os' – into your womb, and take a sample. This is called having a D and C or *dilatation and curettage*. The doctor 'dilates' or stretches the neck of the womb, so he can 'curette' or scrape out a sample or all of the lining of your womb. The surgeon may also make a tiny cut in your stomach, usually near the navel, and pass a narrow periscope-like instrument into your pelvic cavity. This instrument is called a *laparoscope*, and the procedure a *laparoscopy*. The surgeon uses it to peer among the organs all squashed together – your intestines, ovaries, uterus, tubes and bladder.

The level of investigation and the speed with which it is carried out may depend on the symptoms you have when approaching your doctor. What are the diseases or disorders they will be considering?

Identifiable conditions

Cancer

Most women who go to see a doctor for unpleasant symptoms fear that they will be told they have cancer. Cancer is when a group of your own cells begins to grow abnormally. All the cells in your body have specific jobs. Cancer cells have no function, and by taking over from healthy cells stop parts of your body working properly. Some are called benign, a word that usually means friendly. In this case it can be understood as 'innocent'. Benign bundles of cancer cells are covered with a thick skin and remain in one place, growing slowly. Sometimes, they even break down and disappear on their own. These benign tumours can be uncomfortable and a nuisance but it is 'malignant' tumours that cause the real problems. They break up, sending colonies of cells through the body to establish new tumours. This process is called *metastasis*, and the more malignant a tumour, the more likely it is to *metastasize*. To cure cancer, doctors must remove the tumour and make sure no cancerous cells have escaped to set up new colonies elsewhere in your body. You may be given a course of radiation or a 'cytotoxic' or cell-killing drug, or both, to do this.

23

Most hysterectomies are done for reasons other than cancer. So, if a doctor does suggest this operation, do not jump to the conclusion that you have cancer and the doctor isn't telling you so.

Cancer of the cervix
The commonest form of cancer in female reproductive organs is cancer of the cervix – the neck of the womb. More and more women are having smear tests, which is good news for this type of cancer. It has meant that cervical cancer is less likely to get to the point where a hysterectomy is necessary. Cancer of the cervix can be detected at a stage where the cells are just becoming cancerous. At this point they are called *precancerous or non-invasive*. The changes which would make these cells dangerous can take years, and in some cases the body itself can cope. This is why, even though a smear shows some abnormal cells, you may only be asked to return for another test in six to twelve months. At other times, you might be sent to a clinic or hospital to have just the altered cells and the area around them removed. When this is done, healthy cells grow back over the area. Hysterectomy becomes necessary if the cancer cells have developed to the stage when they have become *invasive*. This means that instead of just lying on the surface, affecting skin cells, their effect has spread into the deeper areas and threatens to go further. A symptom of invasive cancer is bleeding at times other than the menstrual period, or of bleeding after the menopause. It often starts as a smelly, brown discharge which can become bright red – especially after making love. This is why any unusual bleeding should *always* be reported to a doctor. Examination and the smear test will usually reveal the problem. You may also be asked to have a *cone biopsy*. This is when the hospital surgeon cuts a small piece out of the cervix, under either local or general anaesthetic, for laboratory testing.

Endometrial cancer
The second most common cancer is endometrial cancer, or cancer of the womb itself. Again, the most important symptom of this is unusual bleeding, which may be brown or foul-smelling.

Occasionally, the growth blocks up the channel from the uterus, so instead of bleeding you might feel feverish and have pain. An ordinary vaginal examination might not show much. You would need to have a D and C 'scrape' for the doctor to see the telltale signs. Sometimes the condition is caught early enough so that it is enough to remove the lining of the womb. This is followed by chemotherapy – a course of certain drugs. More usually, surgery must take away the womb, cervix and other tissue. You would then be given radiation and drug therapy to make sure the cancer did not spread to other organs in your body.

Ovarian cancer
The third most common cancer is of the ovaries. Ovarian cancer is often 'silent'. That is, it gets to quite an advanced stage before you can tell anything is wrong. The cancer cells form a tumour – a swelling – on the ovary. It can grow to quite a size. The first signs of its existence may be that you get a pot belly, as if you were putting on weight or had become pregnant. The tumour can press upon other organs in the pelvic cavity. It can make you want to pass water unusually often or feel as if something was pressing downwards inside you. It can sometimes even cause pain. Most ovarian tumours or cysts are benign. They feel uncomfortable but are unable to spread to other parts of your body or otherwise harm you. A small tumour can be removed, leaving the ovary intact. When the tumour is large, the affected ovary may have to come out, too. Even if this happens, the human body provides two of nearly everything. In time the remaining ovary will take over all functions, leaving you as fertile as before. With a malignant tumour, however, a hysterectomy is usually necessary.

Endometriosis
Your womb is lined with endometrial tissue. Each month, it thickens and is then shed as your menstrual period. Endometriosis is when some of this tissue appears in the pelvic cavity. It can grow on the ovaries, on the outside of the womb, on the Fallopian tubes, the bladder or the intestines, or on the ligaments holding

the uterus in place and walls of the pelvic cavity. If you have had any abdominal operations, it may grow on the scar tissue. Each month, these patches follow the example of the lining of the womb. They build up, and then bleed. Unlike blood in the womb, however, there is nowhere it can go. Small cysts are formed and increase in size every month. They become a dark brown, and so are called 'chocolate cysts'. These cysts can cause scarring or *adhesions*, which stick together affected organs in your pelvic cavity. Endometriosis can be difficult to diagnose. The symptoms are usually pelvic pain, before or sometimes during a period. Periods can be unusually heavy and frequent. You might find making love is uncomfortable, causing a deep ache or stabbing sensation. Opening your bowels may also hurt. A doctor might be able to feel lumps which would be tender, and any attempt to move your womb might also hurt, if the adhesions hold it in place. Endometriosis can make you feel tired, sluggish and depressed. Often, it is not diagnosed until a laparoscopy is performed. Women can suffer pain, discomfort and depression for years before a doctor takes them seriously enough to recommend such an operation. Having been diagnosed, endometriosis can be dealt with by surgery or chemotherapy or a combination of the two. Hormone treatments may be used to either lower the amount of oestrogen in your body or increase the amount of other sex hormones to have a similar effect. There are now quite a variety of treatments available for endometriosis, although it has to be said that this is a difficult condition that medical science is still finding out about.

Pelvic inflammatory disease (PID)

Pelvic inflammatory disease can affect the ovaries, Fallopian tubes and uterus. Infection can be *acute*, where there will be a flare-up of serious symptoms, or *chronic*, where you would feel vaguely ill for some time. PID can follow trauma during childbirth or an induced or natural abortion. Sexually transmitted diseases such as chlamydia or gonorrhoea or non-specific genital infection can also be a cause. Intrauterine contraceptive devices can be associated with infection. Infection can be spread from other diseased organs by the bloodstream or the urinary tract – a burst appendix, for instance. If you had acute PID, the symptoms you would probably notice would be high fever, a smelly vaginal discharge and pain in your abdomen. Chronic PID might give you occasional aching pain, especially during periods and lovemaking, and heavy menstrual bleeding. Pain comes not only from the infection, but from the scar tissue that builds up after an infection and sticks parts of your body such as your tubes, ovaries and uterus together.

If caught in time, PID can be treated with antibiotics and is actually the least common reason for a hysterectomy. Prevention is the key, and a woman at risk of any of the possible causes should be alert to early signs. A prolonged course of antibiotics might be preferable to hysterectomy, but in severe cases, surgery will be the only option.

Fibromyomata (fibroids)

Fibroids are bundles of fibrous tissue that can grow within the muscle of your womb. They are said to affect as many as a quarter of all women and are the most common reason for having a hysterectomy. However, not every woman who has fibroids is troubled by them. They are not dangerous in themselves – they are not cancerous. Fibroids grow singly or in groups and can be as small as a pea or as large as a grapefruit. The typical sites for them to develop are:

- on the outside of the uterus, when they are called subserous fibroids;
- under the endometrium or lining of the womb, when they are called submucous fibroids;
- inside the wall of the uterus, when they are called intramural fibroids.

Types of fibroid

'Subserous fibroids', which grow just under the skin covering the uterus, can grow for some time without giving you any trouble. If they become large, however, they could press against other

27

organs in your pelvic cavity, such as the bowel or bladder. This may make opening your bowels or passing water painful or difficult, or may cause you to want to pass water more often. Sometimes the fibroid grows out on a stalk, wraps around itself and cuts off its own blood supply. You would feel pain which, if left, would eventually stop as the fibroid died. In time, the dead fibroid would become hard and form what used to be known as a 'womb stone'.

'Submucous fibroids' cause the most discomfort. Since they bulge out under the lining of the womb, they stretch and increase its surface area. This means you will lose more blood during your period, which may last longer. You may lose so much extra blood that you become anaemic and feel tired, weak and unwell. Submucous fibroids can also grow stalks extending into the womb. When this happens, the uterus reacts as it would to any unusual 'foreign body' and tries to push it out. You may then suffer painful cramps, especially during your period. Sometimes the uterus succeeds in partly expelling the fibroid and it jams the cervix open, giving you constant pain and bleeding.

'Intramural fibroids' give the least trouble of all. You may only notice them if they grow large enough to give you a pot belly.

Treating fibroids
Some doctors may not want to operate because of fibroids, especially if you are approaching menopause. After menopause, the level of female hormones in your blood will drop and your fibroids will shrink in size. So they may want to 'wait and see', in case the situation clears up on its own. Until this happens, you may be offered iron tablets and possibly a D and C to encourage the lining to come away quickly. Other doctors may be keen to offer a hysterectomy, even when you don't want it, and you may be right to be cautious. Even intramural fibroids, deep in the muscle of the womb, can be removed on their own without having to take away the whole womb. This operation, called a *myomectomy*, 'shells' out the fibroids, and the surgeon then 'nips and tucks' the uterus back into shape. However, if the fibroids are large and numerous, this can be a tricky operation and it can be

difficult to stop the uterus bleeding. Unless there are very good reasons for you to keep your womb, a surgeon may suggest a hysterectomy instead. Even if the surgeon sets off to do a myomectomy, complications may make a hysterectomy necessary.

Prolapse of the womb

A prolapse is when the tissues which support the womb or the vagina become slack. The walls of the vagina then sag inwards under the weight of the rectum or the bladder, or the womb slumps down into the vagina. You may feel a dragging, 'bearing-down' sensation. You may find a lump in the wall of your vagina, which could disappear after lying down or worsen as your bladder fills. You may also suffer from *stress incontinence*, when you lose a few drops or a rush of urine on sneezing or jumping. You might also find that you have to return to the lavatory several times, needing to pass a few more drops you could not squeeze out at the first attempt. Sometimes, the womb drops so far that your cervix can be pushed out of the vagina when you strain. In some cases, prolapse is severe enough to let the whole womb bulge out. This is called a *procidentia*. Prolapse used to be fairly common. It happens when tissue surrounding the womb is stretched and damaged. For example, straining too soon during childbirth, difficult labour or too frequent pregnancies can all increase your chances of suffering one; so will straining of the pelvic muscles too quickly after labour before they have had a chance to heal. Better care for women during pregnancy and labour and after childbirth, as well as smaller families, has meant that prolapse is becoming less common.

Treatment of prolapse

When the prolapse is less severe, a repair operation may be all that is necessary. You would correct a stretched, slack waistband by snipping out a section and joining the edges together. So the surgeon cuts ligaments, muscles and tissue to restore elasticity to your vagina and lift the womb back in place. In some situations, instead of surgery, the womb is gently pushed back into its correct position and is then held in place with a polythene ring. This ring is like a contraceptive diaphragm, but without the covering dome. The device is called a *Hodge Pessary* and it can be taken out, cleaned and replaced regularly.

Disorders

You might ask a doctor for help if your periods have become heavy, frequent or painful. Or it may be because lovemaking has become uncomfortable to painful. Often, the doctor can find no sign of any conditions such as cancer, PID or endometriosis. They then give labels to the *symptoms* you present, as if they themselves were diseases. The broad term often used is *dysfunctional uterine bleeding*, or DUB, or *abnormal uterine bleeding*, or AUB. Both just mean bleeding from the womb for which the doctor can find no good reason.

To be more specific, the doctor may give one of the following names to describe your situation.

Menorrhagia

Menorrhagia means heavy bleeding. The average amount lost during a period is about 70 ml, although some women lose more, some less. Menstrual cycles can vary in length from 21 to 35 days, 28 being an average figure. Whatever the length of your cycle, it will usually be the same from month to month with no more than a two-day difference. If your cycle is less than three weeks long, a doctor would want to investigate. Bleeding between periods, unless it is 'breakthrough bleeding' from being on the Pill, should always be checked out.

Dysmenorrhoea

Dysmenorrhoea simply means period pain. You could have 'primary' or 'secondary' dysmenorrhoea. Primary dysmenorrhoea is when there is no disease or condition to cause the pain. Secondary is when you have a condition such as endometriosis to explain it. Dysmenorrhoea can mean stabbing pains in the lower abdomen, back and inner thighs which strike without warning,

The problems that may lead to having a hysterectomy
(the affected areas are shaded)

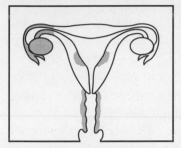

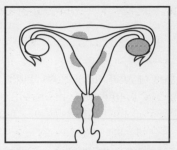

P.I.D. Can affect the Fallopian tubes, ovaries, womb and vagina.

Cancer Can affect the ovaries, lining of the womb (endometrium), cervix and vagina.

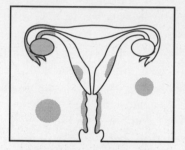

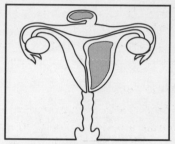

Endometriosis Can affect the ovaries, the Fallopian tubes, the outside of the womb, the pelvic cavity, the bladder and the vagina.

Fibroids Found in the womb – deep within the walls, or just under the outer or inner lining.

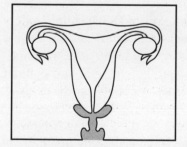

Prolapse

31

fading to a dull ache and then returning. You may find yourself doubled over, and the only comfort can be curling up with a hot water bottle.

Dysmenorrhoea may build up over several days, if not a full week, before your period. Instead of stabbing pains, you may feel a heavy, sickening ache in your lower abdomen, often with headache, backache and pains in the breasts. You may be constipated, lose your appetite and feel tetchy and depressed. Some people find the symptoms clear up as soon as your period starts. Others find they continue throughout a period.

How heavy is a 'heavy' period?

The main difficulty facing you and your doctor is in deciding what is 'heavy' and 'painful' when applied to periods. Studies have shown that women's assessment of their own menstrual loss often varies, one woman considering 70 ml to be a 'light loss' and another that 20 ml is a 'heavy loss'. Pain is also very difficult to measure, one person ignoring an injury which would make another person cry. Unfortunately, it became fashionable during our grandparents' day to insist, against all the evidence, that 'women are the weaker sex'. That, combined with the even older beliefs linking the womb to 'hysterical' behaviour, still influences some doctors so that they cannot take seriously a woman's complaints and description of her symptoms.

Hormone imbalance

Although doctors cannot always explain DUB, it does appear that an imbalance in the hormones – the chemical messengers that control menstruation and ovulation – is likely to be to blame. Too much oestrogen, for instance, and the endometrium or lining of the womb grows thicker than usual. A period may be delayed, but be heavier and longer than before. Too little progesterone and the lining is thin and comes away early, causing frequent and prolonged periods. Period pain can be caused by the lining of the womb producing substances called *prostaglandins*. These are natural chemicals which cause the muscles in the uterine wall to contract, forcing out period blood and tissue. But too many of them leads to cramps.

Before even considering a hysterectomy for DUB, you and your doctor would want to try to control the underlying reason for your symptoms. Female hormones – oestrogen, progestogen, synthetic progesterone or a combination of the antiprostaglandin drugs – may correct the imbalance. Your doctor may give you combined oestrogen and progestogen in the form of the combined contraceptive pill, to be taken every night for three out of every four weeks. Or you may be prescribed the progestogen-only pill, to be taken every night, or for two weeks, of each month. You may be given a drug called clomiphene, to try and get your pituitary gland to work and produce its own hormones. If your main symptom is painful cramps, a non-steroidal anti-inflamma- tory drug (NSAID) such as mefenamic acid (Ponstan) or ibuprofen or aspirin may be suggested, as all block the release of prostaglandins. After a six-month course of hormones, you may find that menstruation has returned to normal. If not, your doctor may want to send you for a D and C before discussing the next step. This is often suggested as, in itself, a D and C can sometimes clear up painful, heavy periods. However, there is evidence that it only does so for a short time. Heavy and painful periods may return, so it might only be a delaying tactic.

What are the likely reasons for this imbalance in hormones? Being underweight or overweight can have this effect. So, rather than advise drug or hormone treatment, your doctor might start off suggesting that you adjust your diet. The doctor may also recommend regular and energetic exercise. If you smoke, you may also be advised to stop, since the nicotine in tobacco has an effect on muscles. Heavy smoking during period pains might make you feel calmer, but it could actually increase the cramps. You might also find that you are asked about your feelings and whether anything is worrying you. In doing this, a doctor would not be hinting that your problems are 'all in the mind' or that you are being neurotic. The myth that there is a link between the womb and the emotions has some truth, in that stress can affect the production of hormones. This is why women often find their periods arrive early or late during an upheaval – moving house, starting a new job, going on holiday or any important event. Problems with your periods could be your body's way of signalling that something is troubling you about your life. If this were so, it would be better to tackle the cause itself than remove your womb.

The IUS

One treatment for menorrhagia or heavy bleeding that is having significant and exciting results is the intrauterine system, or IUS. This is a small plastic device which is put into the womb. The IUS (trade name Mirena) releases a steady amount of progestogen. It was originally developed as a method of birth control. But women who used the IUS found it reduced period blood loss by as much as 90 per cent. It also has few side-effects. In one study, 82 per cent of women who used the IUS found it helped their heavy bleeding so much they came off the waiting list for a hysterectomy. Many GPs are now suggesting an IUS as first treatment for heavy bleeding. When women come to them who might once have been sent for a D and C or a hysterectomy, now the idea is to try the IUS to see if it helps. Once in place, the device can be left and is effective, for treatment and as birth control, for up to five years.

Endometrial ablation and resection

A D and C, by removing the lining of the womb for the time being, may in itself clear up the problem. More often, it offers temporary relief and the problem comes back. Where bleeding is the problem and there are no other reasons for having to remove the womb, there is something that can be done before the drastic step of a hysterectomy. This is endometrial ablation or resection. Endometrial resection is when the inner lining of the womb is destroyed. Endometrial ablation destroys the entire lining. Heavy bleeding can often be stopped or greatly reduced, but you won't be able to go through a pregnancy afterwards. The lining of the womb is removed with a laser or by reaming it away with a wire loop or curved blade, or burned away with a heated roller

34

ball. As the loop or blade cuts away, an electrical current is passed through it to seal the tissue as it goes. When tissue is heat sealed by laser or electric current, the lining will not grow again, so you are left with your womb intact but no more periods. A new form of endometrial ablation uses microwave energy. Microwaves in microwave ovens heat up food all the way through. Microwaves used for endometrial ablation only go 6 mm into tissue – enough to heat up and destroy the lining but not enough to harm any further. Endometrial ablation with microwave energy is very simple. It takes three to five minutes on average, can be done under local anaesthesia and patients require fewer painkillers after. Early studies have shown that the problem bleeding rate after endometrial ablation with microwave energy is much less than with other methods. The advantages of endometrial ablation and resection over hysterectomy are that it can be done in a day or with an overnight stay. It can be done under local anaesthesia and there are no scars. Since the ovaries are untouched, you don't get hot flushes or mood changes afterwards. But you will need to go on having normal smear tests. The disadvantage is that in some cases periods do come back.

Your relationship with your doctor

Some doctors are unsympathetic. If they themselves have never experienced a bad period, or have been brought up to consider 'female problems' something that every woman has to suffer, preferably in silence, you may have difficulty in getting a fair hearing. However, be careful that you do not dismiss painful home truths as lack of understanding. If you are convinced that your doctor is being less than helpful, remember that you do have the right to ask for a second opinion. Your doctor can choose whether to send you to another general practitioner – another member of a partnership, for instance – or to a hospital doctor. If the second is as unhelpful as the first, you *can* change general practitioners without having to give an explanation. Ask around your friends for a good one, go along to their surgery, if possible with your medical card, and request that you be taken on to the list. All you then have to do is sign a form and wait two weeks before seeing your new doctor.

Whether you will be referred for hysterectomy or given alternative treatment will be the decision of your doctor and the hospital surgeon who would perform the operation. But it is *your* body and *your* symptoms that are under discussion. You have every right to insist on an explanation from your doctors. You are not being 'difficult' or 'wasting their time' to ask why your difficulties are happening, what their investigations reveal and how their treatment will affect you. Ultimately, no one can force you to have an operation you are not satisfied is necessary, or continue treatment that is uncomfortable or ineffectual. *Remember that!* Similarly, *you* cannot insist that a doctor prescribes treatment you consider correct. Ideally, the relationship between patient and doctor is one of mutual trust and respect, with both sides being able to explain to each other what is happening and to listen to and accept each other's statements. Sadly, too many doctors still feel that the 'perfect patient' is passive, asking no questions and taking no part in their own cure. You may find some doctors feel challenged and threatened if you step out of this traditional role. While it might be satisfying to let them know in no uncertain terms where you think you both stand, it will not help you if you are thrown out of the clinic!

Questions to ask

Before you say yes to a hysterectomy, you might like to ask yourself the following questions:

- Do I still want to become pregnant?
- Is the possibility of becoming pregnant important to me – does it make me feel 'feminine'?
- Do we know what is causing my symptoms?
- Are the symptoms bad enough to interfere with my everyday life?
- Is the condition serious enough to threaten my health?
- Have we tried every other treatment for my problem?

- Am I happy about having a hysterectomy and sure that it will solve my problems?
- Am I satisfied that I do not need another medical opinion?

If you find yourself saying yes to either of the first two questions and no to any of the others, it would be a good idea to talk to your doctor. Clearly, you need either an opportunity to talk about your feelings, more information or a stab at alternative treatments.

In the next chapter, we will consider what happens if your answers and your doctor's advice mean the operation *is* for you.

5

The Different Operations for Hysterectomy

I'd expected all sorts of things to happen to me after my hysterectomy – hot flushes, that sort of thing. When I mentioned it to my GP, he said, 'Ah, but you've only had a total hysterectomy, they left you your ovaries.' I was confused, to say the least. I remember saying to him, 'But I thought that's what a hysterectomy meant, having them taken away? What do you mean, *only* a total hysterectomy?'

Sarah W

We are actually being rather vague when we talk about 'having a hysterectomy', because there are four types of this operation. There are also two ways of getting into your body to do it. The surgeon can cut through your abdomen or stomach wall to reach the pelvic cavity, or go through the vagina. The route chosen depends on the type of hysterectomy that must be done. And *that* depends on the medical condition from which you are suffering. Your surgeon can:

- remove the womb only. This is called a *subtotal hysterectomy*.
- remove the womb and the cervix. This is called a *total hysterectomy.*
- remove the womb, cervix, both Fallopian tubes and the ovaries. This is called a *total hysterectomy with bilateral salpingo-oophorectomy.*
- remove the womb, cervix, both Fallopian tubes and ovaries, the upper part of the vagina and ligaments, lymph glands and fatty tissue from the pelvic cavity. This is called *extended* or *Wertheim's hysterectomy.*

The different operations, and what is removed in each (the area removed is shaded)

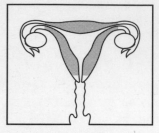

Sub-total Womb only.

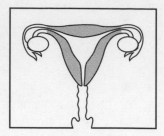

Total Womb and cervix.

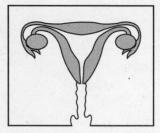

Total, with bi-lateral salpingo-oophorectomy Womb, cervix, Fallopian tubes and ovaries.

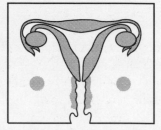

Wertheim Womb, cervix, Fallopian tubes, ovaries, part of the vagina and lymph nodes.

You may hear the last two operations referred to by your doctors as a *pelvic clearance*. You must remember that your uterus, ovaries and tubes do not float around in a hollow in the middle of your body. All these organs are held in place by a network of ligaments, and squashed together with other organs – coils of intestine, your bladder and rectum. Veins and arteries carry blood to and from every organ. Performing an operation is a demanding and exhausting job, both physically and emotionally. Not only must the surgeon and assistants cut through tough flesh and ligaments, and push aside and lift out heavy organs, they must also be constantly on the look-out. In a diagram, it seems simple to work out which tube is which. When you are peering into a mass of tissue and blood, it is not so easy. No surgeon *should* cut through one of your ureters – the tubes carrying your urine from kidneys to bladder – or harm your bowel. But it can, if rarely, happen. If you were to see what the surgeon is faced with when he opens up your body, such mistakes would be more understandable. By the time the surgeon is ready to lift out your womb, your pelvic cavity is likely to resemble a jar full of cutlery! You will be full of clamps to hold your abdomen open, your arteries closed and your organs steady. So when choosing the best hysterectomy operation for you, these considerations will play a small part in the decision.

Subtotal hysterectomy

Subtotal hysterectomies are rarely done these days. It used to be a popular operation because it is quick and easy and the woman loses very little blood. But it leaves the cervix a potential site for cancer. You would still have to have regular smear tests and may well end up having to have the cervix removed at some time in the future anyway. Nowadays, a surgeon would only do a subtotal if the more extended operation would put you at risk. Extensive scar tissue, after endometriosis for instance, might make it difficult. In cutting away the scar tissue, your bowel and bladder could be in the way and be damaged. Subtotal hysterectomy may be the choice, then, when the uterus alone has been affected and operating difficulties limit the surgeon's movements.

Total hysterectomy

More often you would be offered a total hysterectomy. In reality, this operation is far from 'total'. It removes the womb and the cervix but it leaves your ovaries. It is the ovaries that produce the bulk of female hormones every month. The ovaries are driven on by the pituitary gland, which is at the base of the brain. Total hysterectomy is the choice when fibroids, endometriosis, prolapse or period problems have led to an operation being necessary, but your ovaries are unaffected. After the operation, the ovaries will continue to work and, in the main, you will feel no different. Sometimes, one or part of an ovary will have been involved and need to be removed. Within a few months, the remaining ovarian tissue will have adapted and taken over the job once done by both ovaries.

Without functioning ovaries, a woman enters the menopause. The loss of natural oestrogen produced by her ovaries can give rise to a wide range of troubling symptoms. You may experience 'hot flushes', when your face and neck blush a bright red and you break out in a sweat. You may feel dizzy and your heart may race. Some women suffer 'formication' (watch how you pronounce that – it has an 'm', not an 'n', in the middle!). This is a curious itching feeling, as if ants were crawling under your skin – hence the name, from the Latin for ants. Some women suffer depression, headaches, insomnia, loss of memory and concentration, tiredness or irritability as a result of the menopause. You can also find your skin drying out and becoming more wrinkled. Your vagina can become less elastic and moist, making penetrative sex painful. You could suffer from cystitis – an irritation in the urinary tract or water passage – and find yourself wanting to pass water frequently. Lack of oestrogen also means your bones lose calcium and become thinner and far more likely to snap. All this is why doctors may do their best to leave you at least one ovary if you are having a hysterectomy before you have entered your natural menopause.

Total hysterectomy with bilateral salpingo-oophorectomy

If you have the operation after the menopause, however, your ovaries will be removed for the same reason as the cervix – just in case they cause trouble in the future. So, a total hysterectomy with bilateral salpingo-oophorectomy (or both-sided Fallopian tube and ovary removal) will be done when a woman is past her menopause. It will also be the choice when the operation is for a condition that affects the ovaries and/or tubes as well as the womb. Such a condition could be large fibroids, cancer in the uterus or ovaries, extensive endometriosis or pelvic inflammatory disease (PID).

In the bad old days, such an operation meant a premature menopause for many women. All the frightening myths about hysterectomy – that it makes you old, fat, hairy and means the end of your sex life – date from this. The menopause does not always have this effect, but it can make life uncomfortable and difficult. However, these days, the removal of your ovaries need mean nothing of the sort. If your ovaries were still working, most doctors will automatically prescribe oestrogen for you, to replace the oestrogen no longer made in your body. This hormone replacement therapy, or HRT, is taken as tablets by mouth, as a patch to be stuck on the skin, or as an implant slipped under the skin of your stomach or buttock. Current research shows that HRT has more benefits than risks. There seems to be a very slight increase in breast cancer among women using HRT for more than five years. This is similar to the slightly increased risk for women using thc Pill for such a time. You do need to balance that up against the other conditions it protects against, such as heart disease and osteoporosis, both of which can kill. And the breast cancers that are found tend to be slower growing and less invasive. The important point is that any woman on hormone therapy needs to have regular medical check-ups and do her own breast checks. And you should be doing that anyway! In the long run, HRT protects you more than it puts you at risk.

The main cancer that might be increased by HRT is cancer of the endometrium. Women who have not had a hysterectomy and are taking oestrogen on its own for the symptoms of natural menopause can have an increased risk. This is not a problem if progestogen is given as well. Since after a hysterectomy you will no longer have an endometrium, this need not worry you. Properly prescribed HRT would mean that a hysterectomy that removes your functioning ovaries would have the same effects on you as one that left them in place. Oestrogen therapy may not be possible for some women. In this case, your doctor could offer a variety of treatments to help with menopausal symptoms if and as they arose.

ed or Wertheim's hysterectomy

peration is for cancer that has become invasive and
tening to spread, you may well have an extended or
Wertheim's hysterectomy. An extended hysterectomy removes
your womb, tubes, ovaries, cervix and the top of the vagina. A
Wertheim's goes even further, paring away the upper two-thirds
of the vagina and the fatty tissue and lymph glands in the pelvis
into which the cancer cells may have migrated. Needless to say,
this is quite extensive surgery.

Surgical procedure

Your surgeon can choose to go through the vagina or the
abdomen to reach your womb for the operation. Each method has
its advantages and disadvantages. A vaginal hysterectomy would
leave you with no visible scar and less 'trauma'. Your body
obviously reacts with shock when muscle and tissue are cut open.
The vaginal route makes sense when the surgeon only has to
remove womb and cervix, especially when both have already
advanced into the passage, such as in a prolapse. In this situation,
the surgeon would also be wanting to repair slack tissue in this
area and so would do it all at once. The drawbacks of a vaginal
hysterectomy are that the wound has a slightly higher risk of
bleeding and becoming infected. The operation does require more
skill than if done through the abdominal wall. Coming from
below you, the surgeon has less opportunity to have a good look
round the pelvic cavity and check on the health of all the other
organs. Also, a vaginal wound may shorten and narrow the end of
the vagina. In some cases, two small cuts are made, one by your
navel and another at the bikini line. The surgical team can insert a
laparoscope in the navel cut, so they can have a clearer picture of
what they are doing. They can also insert some instruments in the
bikini cut, to help the operation.

In most cases, the surgeon will want to open your abdomen to
operate. You will probably have a bikini cut, called a Pfannensteil
incision after the doctor who perfected it. This is a horizontal cut

across your belly, just below your pubic hair line. As the name suggests, it should be invisible even when you wear a bikini. If your womb is especially enlarged by fibroids, or you have a large cyst on an ovary, the surgeon may have to make a vertical cut down the midline of your belly. This leaves a wound which takes longer to heal than the bikini cut. But, if your surgeon needs to use it, there will be a good reason.

With the removal of your womb and whatever other organs had to go, you are not left with a hollow in the middle of your body. In their natural state, remember, your womb, ovaries and tubes were only the size of a large pear and a couple of plums. If swollen by cysts or fibroids, they would have been pushing other organs aside to make room. Once gone, your bladder and intestines will gladly shuffle around and take up the space! Nor will you have a hole leading from the top of your vagina into the cavity. During the operation, your surgeon will sew up the gap left by the removal of the cervix. In some circumstances, the hole is left partially open to allow for drainage, closing and healing on its own after a few weeks. Otherwise, it is stitched closed at once.

When it is decided that you will have a hysterectomy, discuss with your doctor the sort of operation you will be having and the route that will be taken. You might like to make a note of the type of operation so that you will know in the future what has been taken out and what left. Knowing which type, and which incision will be made, gives you a chance to prepare yourself for what will happen once you go into hospital.

6

Going into Hospital

It wasn't the operation itself that frightened me. It was going into hospital! Hospitals make me nervous – all those doctors and nurses – you never know who anyone is or what they want of you. I was in a spin from beginning to end, totally confused. I kept thinking, 'I hope they know what's going on, because I certainly don't!'

Vera S

Having seen the hospital doctor and decided between you that you will be going in for a hysterectomy, what then? You will be put on a waiting list, and how quickly you will be called in for the operation may depend on your state of health and the size of that list. If your doctor fears that you have a metastasizing carcinoma – cancer that is spreading – you are likely to be given an immediate date. With fibroids that are giving you only moderate pain, you may have to hang around for months. Waiting time can vary from hospital to hospital. Large city teaching hospitals often have longer waiting lists than those in small country towns. Having kicked your heels for a time, you will probably receive a letter giving you a few weeks' notice. Very occasionally, you might get a phone call asking you to come in with only a few hours' or a day's warning. This would only happen if someone else had cancelled their operation, and rather than leave the bed and operating time empty, the hospital admissions staff try to fill it. This may be inconvenient. But saying yes could allow you to have your operation weeks or months ahead of when you otherwise might have had it. It may also be possible to have your doctor refer you outside your immediate area to a hospital with a shorter waiting list. If you are willing to travel, discuss this with your doctor.

The thought of going into hospital unnerves most people. After all, hospitals are linked in our minds with illness and death. The unmistakable smell of hospital disinfectant makes many of us feel sick and shaky. Smells and colours have a powerful ability to bring back painful memories – or just the pain without the clear memory! If you are frightened, don't feel silly or unusual. You'll be in the *majority*. If you confess your feelings to your friends and family, the medical staff and other patients, you'll probably find they will share your feelings, understand and sympathize.

Early preparation before going into hospital

There are four important steps you might need to take before going into hospital, to make your stay more comfortable.

Stop smoking

Lots of people get chest infections after an operation. It is a common side-effect and doesn't happen because the hospital has failed to look after you properly. But the risks of your getting a chest infection are far, far greater if you smoke. Trying to cough up loads of sticky fluid while you have stitches in your tummy is far from amusing. You will need to be off cigarettes for at least a fortnight before your admission to see any benefit. So you may as well begin to quit as soon as you know you are to have the operation.

Stop taking the Pill

If you are using oral contraception, you will need to finish a month or so before your operation and use another method until you go into hospital. This is because the Pill increases your chances of suffering a blood clot during or after the operation. If yours is a sudden admission, remind the doctor that you were on the Pill. You may be given treatment to thin your blood or have a special watch kept on your condition.

Get fit

If you don't do it already, start taking exercise. Walk briskly, swim, run or cycle most days. Or join a fitness class two to three times a week. If you have problems with movement, talk to your doctor. You may find special help in your area for anyone who wants to get fit and has difficulties. Your doctor will be happy to back you. The fitter you are when you go into hospital, the quicker you will recover.

Get organized!

While you are in hospital, the only person you should be thinking and worrying about is yourself. Wondering whether your family or your work colleagues can manage without you will not help you recover quickly. If your immediate family cannot cook and clean for themselves, make sure you leave a well-stocked fridge or freezer and fix up support among friends, neighbours and other family members. Better still, give them a crash course on looking after themselves, and you, before you go in. You will not make yourself redundant by teaching a husband or son to cook or iron for themselves – they love and need you as more than a housekeeper. Also, they are going to have to look after *you* for some time after you come home – they may as well start practising now.

What to take with you

The night before admission, pack your bag. You will be in hospital for between five and ten days. While visitors can bring you various forgotten items, you will find the first few days easier if you take the following with you.

Essential clothing

Hospitals can lend you dressing-gowns and night-gowns, so if you are used to sleeping in the buff, you do not have to spend money on clothes just for this visit. You might feel happier, however, in your own things – T-shirt and pants or leggings are fine, if that's what you prefer. You will want at least one change of nightwear. You may also want a dressing-gown or robe and slippers. You might also like a top, shawl or jacket to wear while sitting up in bed.

Toilet things

You will need toothpaste and brush, hairbrush and/or comb and a flannel or sponge. The hospital can provide soap, but your own favourite soap, talcum powder, shampoo and deodorant will be a morale booster. So will make-up. Taking nail scissors, files, hand cream and nail polish will give you the chance to give yourself a manicure, too. You also need some sanitary *pads*, not tampons, to use after the operation.

Entertainment and contact

You will need something to while away the time waiting for the next doctor to see you, friends to visit, cup of tea to arrive or stitches to come out. Take reading material – books and magazines. This may be the time to get through *War and Peace*, but remember, you might need something light and easy, too. Take notepaper, stamps and pen and catch up on overdue letters. Also make sure you have a supply of coins or a charge card for the phone, and the phone numbers of family and friends. Hospitals don't let you use a mobile as it can interfere with sensitive machinery. Most hospitals offer 'piped' radio and headphones, and some even have their own radio station. The number of channels may be limited, though, so you might like to take your own radio, or a cassette or CD player (don't forget to take headphones!). You can even take your own portable television, with the same provision. You might like some photos of your family, to cheer you up.

Money and valuables

You will want a bit of money for phone calls and newspapers. You can give anything of value you have to bring with you to the nursing staff for safe keeping.

Documents

Bring your appointment card and the letter from the hospital. If you are on social security or a pension, bring the books too.

Your letter will tell you where you should present yourself – at the ward or at the Admissions Office. Wherever you start, the routine is roughly the same – and just as tedious and irritating! You will be asked to give details such as name, address and age, for the twenty-seventh time. Try not to be annoyed; it is better to give your name once too often than end up on the wrong operating table. You will have a plastic bracelet with your name and age, and the name of your surgeon, fastened to your wrist. However ugly and absurd you think it looks, do not even *think* of taking it off. This is your guarantee that it is your womb and not your spleen, appendix or right leg that will be removed. At some point in this procedure, you will be taken to your ward, introduced to the sister in charge and given a bed.

Be choosy about the possessions you bring. You'll only have a small bedside cabinet and bed table, which can get cluttered.

Staff you will meet

Nurses

The *sister* is the first of many medical and other hospital staff you are likely to see quite regularly over the next week or so. He or she is in charge of your ward and everything that goes on in it. Under them, there is a team of nurses. There will be at least one *staff nurse* – usually called 'staff' for short. These are Registered Nurses (RNs), who trained to diploma or degree level. Below them are RN students, in their first, second or third years of training. In some large wards there may be a *senior staff nurse* or a *junior sister* or *charge nurse*. There will also be *nursing auxiliaries*, to help bathe or wash you and organize non-medical routine on the ward. Hospitals have their own uniforms – dress or belt colours or shoulder tabs and badges to show who is who. Nurses are often proud of their rank, so give them a chance to show off and orientate yourself by asking!

Doctors

The doctors you will see are grouped in what is known as a 'firm'. Head of this is the *consultant*, a specialist of many years' experience in gynaecological obstetrics. Under him or her is a team of so-called 'junior' doctors – although they are far from junior in most senses of the word. Under the consultant is usually

51

a *registrar* and then one or two *senior house officers*. They are all in training to become consultants themselves and are often just waiting for a vacancy to come up. Below them are *house officers*. They are also sometimes called housemen – confusing if, as is more and more likely nowadays, they happen to be women! A house officer is a fully qualified doctor, so do not let the 'junior' title make you feel as if you are in the hands of someone who does not know their job. In a teaching hospital, the 'firm' will have a group of medical students. They may observe your treatment but would only be asked to do anything themselves under strict supervision. As well as these people, you will come into contact with laboratory technicians who may take blood from you, physiotherapists who help you get over your operation, and hospital porters and cleaning staff and volunteers who make your stay more pleasant.

After admission

Having shown you to your bed, a nurse will complete all the paperwork and move on to a long list of medical checks. You will be asked to undress, and the nurse will take your pulse, temperature and blood pressure. This is all recorded on a chart which will probably be hung on the end of your bed. You will also be asked to give a urine or water specimen. The operation itself will not take place until at least the following day. Sometimes, you will even be asked to come in two or three days in advance. There are good reasons for this. Before you can be given the final all-clear for the operation, a doctor must make sure you are in good health. A junior doctor, probably a house officer, will see you, and give you a thorough medical check-up. Blood and other tests may need to be done, and they can take a day or two to come back from the laboratory. The delay will give you a chance to relax and wind down. If there are any doubts about your fitness – if your blood pressure is high, you are 'chesty' or have been taking any medication the doctor feels unhappy about – the *anaesthetist* may be asked to come and see you as well. Some anaesthetists make a routine check on many of the people they will operate on. The anaesthetist is the man or woman who keeps you not only asleep but also alive and breathing during the operation. He or she is the expert on whether you are 'up to' the strain of having an operation. Remember that operation deaths are *very* rare in this country, less than one in every 40,000 operations. So you really have nothing to fear.

Many hospitals now have a sensible routine of asking all patients who are not actually on bed-rest to take their meals together at a table in the ward. Or you may be in a small enough ward that you can talk from your bed with everyone. This gives you an excellent chance to get to know your fellow patients. It's a good idea to make a point of going round and introducing yourself. You will find the support of women who are in the same situation very comforting. If you do feel awkward about asking the doctors and nurses questions, you will find someone in the group prepared to be a spokesperson or give you the encouragement to ask yourself.

At some point, your consultant will make his or her rounds and see you. It is quite possible, on the other hand, that even though your outpatient's appointment card and your hospital records all say you are Mr or Mrs So-and-So's patient, you never actually see them. It could be a registrar who agrees the operation and actually operates on you. But do not feel that you have been fobbed off with second best if this happens. The registrar will be an experienced surgeon too.

Consent forms

As part of the paperwork on your admission, or when you have been pronounced fit to go to the operating theatre, or on the day of your operation itself, you will be asked to sign a consent form. This is a legal document, so read it carefully before giving your signature. The form will say something to this effect:

I, Jane Smith, of 1 The Avenue, Newtown, hereby consent to the operation of total hysterectomy, the nature and the effects of which have been explained to me by Dr Houseman. I also consent to such further measures as may be found necessary during the operation. No assurance has been given to me that the operation will be performed by a particular surgeon.

Make sure that it is your name and address, and that you *do* understand which operation is listed here. If you have any doubts, do not sign until Dr Houseman has explained it to you. The 'further measures' clause is there just in case your surgeon finds something dangerous and unexpected when you are opened up. It would be silly to have to sew you up, bring you round and ask for another signature if you were found to have a badly damaged ovary and had only signed for a 'total'. This does *not* give the surgeon *carte blanche* to go wild, since he or she would have to justify what they thought was 'necessary'. However, you do have the right to strike out this clause if you wish. Talk it over with the doctor.

'Nil by mouth'

Twelve hours before your operation is scheduled, the nurse will hang a 'nil by mouth' sign on your bed. From then until after the operation, *you must not swallow anything*. This is not a piece of silly hospital routine. Ignore it, and you will get more than just a hand slapped. If you are caught out eating or drinking, your operation will be cancelled. If you are not caught you may die. The point is that, while you are under the anaesthetic, if there is food in your stomach your body might throw it out. Vomit on the operating table, and you may choke to death. Or you may inhale, and give yourself serious pneumonia. If that sign is up and anybody gives you something to eat or drink by mistake, do not assume they know what they are doing. They might – your operation could have been set back a few hours – but ask a nurse to check. And *do not* give in to temptation and nibble fruit or sweets. If you are dying of thirst, ask a nurse for a mouthwash. *But do not swallow.*

Shaving

What most people feel is the most embarrassing and uncomfortable preparation for an operation comes next. A nurse will arrive with soap and a razor, and she or you will shave the area where the surgeon will make the incision. In the old days, operation sites were cleared for miles around! The surgical expression was 'from nipples to knees' for any operation in the middle of your body. Nowadays, you need only shave from the top of your pubic hair down to the cleft, if you are having a bikini cut. As well as the soft down on your stomach, the nurse will tell you how much pubic hair you will have to remove if you are having a vertical cut. The reasons you will be asked to shave are twofold. First, hair can hide bacteria, even if you have washed thoroughly. The theatre nurse will swab your skin with disinfectant before the surgeon makes the incision. They will want to be sure a thick growth of hair does not shield even a tiny bit of skin from being thoroughly cleaned. Second, hair will get in the way when it comes to stitching you up.

A few studies have pointed out that skin defuzzed with hair-removing or depilatory cream is even less likely to lead to wound infection than shaving. You might like to get some of the gentle, facial-quality cream from a chemist and use that instead of the razor. Make sure you wash it off thoroughly. Depilated hair grows back with far less itching and discomfort than shaved hair. However, take very great care not to let the cream touch the mucous membranes or soft tissue of your genitals. Or, if you can bear it, you could have a really low bikini wax. Have it done a few days before you go in, so the skin recovers and you can make sure all the wax is washed off.

Elastic stockings

Hospitals now give elastic stockings to patients about to have operations. A period in bed following a major operation can put you at risk of developing dangerous blood clots in your legs. Wearing snugly fitting elastic stockings for the rest of your hospital stay will cut your risks by a significant amount. The support they give encourages blood to circulate and not to pool and stagnate in one part of your leg. However hot and uncomfortable they make you feel, keep these on at all times until the nursing staff tell you it is safe to remove them.

'Premed'

A couple of hours or so before the operation, you will be asked to clear your bowels. This is to prevent you having an 'accident' on the operating table, and to make it easier for the surgeon to move around inside your pelvic cavity. Full intestines would get in the way. It is also in case the surgeon did make a mistake and cut into your bowel. This would cause far more problems if there was waste matter there to spill out into your body. You may be given a suppository or an enema. A nurse will give you a suppository, which is a tampon of gel to gently push into your rectum or back passage. Do it in the lavatory and hold on as long as possible. Or they may use an enema, which is a large syringe (no needles!), to gently flush liquid into you. In a few moments, your bowels will open thoroughly. You will then be asked to have a bath, remove *all* make-up and jewellery, put on a hospital operating gown and relax in bed.

With an hour or so to go, you will be given a 'premed'. This injection has two functions. First, it puts you on cloud nine! It contains a powerful sedative, which makes you relaxed and dozy. Instead of feeling more and more nervous as the time approaches, you may well drift off to sleep. The jab also dries up the saliva in your mouth, nose and throat, so you won't choke on your own spit during the operation. When your turn comes, the hospital porters will arrive at your bedside, expertly and discreetly lift you on to their trolley, and wheel you off to the theatre. A nurse from your ward is likely to come down with you and stay at your side until you are asleep. If this isn't hospital policy and you would like the reassurance of a familiar face, ask to be accompanied to the theatre.

There you will be met by the anaesthetist, who will probably check yet again that you are Mrs Jane Smith (correct him or her if you are not!). Having looked at your medical notes, the anaesthetist will then slide a needle into the back of your hand or your forearm. As the plunger is pressed in, you will feel waves of dizziness sweep across your brain and you will pass out. Your hysterectomy operation is about to begin.

7

After the Operation

The first few days after my hysterectomy were awful. I'd
expected the stitches to hurt – but the fact that I'd still be
having vaginal bleeding took me by surprise and frightened me
at first. I thought something had gone wrong. Then I had a
water infection and I was sure that they'd done something
wrong to allow that to happen. I kept popping to the loo for a
quiet weep, and it really got me down. One of the other women
on the ward was a character – always joking. After a few days,
she got us all talking, and when we found that most of us had
the same problems and we all felt the same, it made such a
difference.

Norma D

You may feel quite surprised when you come round after your
operation, and wonder if it really has happened yet. Unlike
ordinary sleep, the deep blackout you get when under an
anaesthetic gives you no sense of time passing. Many people
come round after an op and are convinced they dozed off and
have woken before going into theatre. They are amazed to find it
is all over. However, you will have been 'out' for between one
and two hours, depending on how quickly your surgeon likes to
work. During this time, your body was draped in green cloths,
leaving just the operation site revealed. Your head and face
would usually have been screened off from the operating team,
and your anaesthetist would have sat by you, watching all the
time to make sure you breathed properly and stayed unconscious.
Some surgeons like to operate to the strains of music – you might
like to find out whether your womb was removed to the sounds of
a Mozart opera, jazz or George Michael! When the last stitch has
been put in, the anaesthetist will start bringing you round. You
will be taken to a 'recovery room', where a nurse will call your
name to see if you respond, and check your pulse and blood
pressure. You will still be light-headed and probably won't be

able to collect your thoughts until you are back in your bed on the ward. Don't be afraid that you might have blurted out any secrets, by the way. It's a myth that anaesthesia acts as a 'truth drug'.

What you will find when you wake up

The 'drip'

A nurse may give you a refreshing and soothing face wash, and could offer you a cup of tea. You will probably drift in and out of sleep for an hour or two. When you finally wake up and take stock, this is what you are likely to find. You may have a 'shunt' in the back of your hand or inside your elbow. This is a needle passed into a vein and taped securely in place. A rubber tube connects this to a drip. This is a plastic bottle hanging over your bed, and a solution of water with salt or salt and sugar (saline and glucose or dextrose) drips slowly into your vein. You will have had a drip going during your operation, to keep you from being dehydrated or dried out. The general anaesthetic and the rummaging about inside your pelvic cavity will have affected your bowels. You may feel sick and will certainly be unable to handle food. Even a drink may make you vomit, so the drip keeps you nourished until you are able to sip liquids. In some cases you may also be given painkilling drugs through a drip or shunt. If you have lost blood, or were anaemic before the operation, the plastic bottle will contain blood instead of water.

The catheter

You may also have a catheter in place. This is a slim tube which goes from your water passage to a collecting bottle or bag. You will have had one inserted during the operation, and it may be left in place for a day or so. You may well develop a urinary infection such as cystitis during this time. This *will not* be because the catheter was dirty or put in clumsily. The very act of operating on this area can cause bruising and make the area delicate. Even a sterile catheter can let in bacteria. This is what triggers the cystitis. You will be tested for any infection and given treatment for it. When the catheter is removed, you may find the muscles around the opening refuse to work at first. You can have a painfully full bladder, but be unable to pass water and so have to have a catheter in again for a further few days. You might like to try a little self-help, though. If you have ever watched cats with their kittens or dogs with puppies, you will know that animals apply a little gentle massage to persuade their young to pass water. While sitting on your bedpan, commode or lavatory, gently rub around the water passage with your fingers. This soothing encouragement may persuade the waters to flow. If you do have an infection, be very careful and ask for some antiseptic jelly or cream to make it easier.

The 'drain'

When the dressing over your scar is changed, you may also find a thin piece of plastic tubing sticking through it. This is a 'drain' and is there to allow fluid to ooze out. As you gradually heal up inside, the fluid will stop coming out and the nurses will eventually pull out the drain. The tiny hole it leaves will close and heal by itself. You may well be pot-bellied with air; this will go down after a few days. You might also have a *haematoma*. This is just a medical term for a large or lumpy bruise, which can be tender. It can be left to drain away by itself and be absorbed by the body like any normal bruise. Or it might leak through your operation wound. Or the doctor might gently probe through the skin and let the blood ooze out.

Discharges

You are likely to find a discharge coming from your vagina. The nurses would have put a sanitary pad between your legs after the operation. If you have not brought your own, they will keep you supplied with clean changes as necessary. The discharge will probably be a reddish-brown. If it becomes bright red, or there are blood clots, or if it turns yellow and smelly, *tell the nurse at once*. About one in every thousand women have a secondary haemorrhage after the operation. This is when the wound in the vagina opens and bleeds. If this happens to you, you might have to rest in bed for an extra day or so, and may need a blood transfusion. Discharges usually stop a fortnight after the operation, although in some cases they can go on for six weeks. Use a pad, not tampons, as these could encourage infections.

In the first few days, the discharge could also be streaked with *blue*. This does not mean you have royal connections your parents never told you about! To make it easier to line up incisions and see how far they have cut, surgeons paint the inside of your vagina with a dye called 'Bonney's blue'. You may find traces of this coming out for some days.

Early days after the operation

How will you feel when you have fully woken up? The area around the operation site will probably feel bruised and painful. You are likely to be offered painkillers. There is no point in being brave, so do not refuse these, and tell a nurse if you feel uncomfortable between drug rounds. You may feel 'chesty' and want to cough. This is a good idea, to help clear your lungs and stop a chest infection. You will find it easier to cough if you sit up, bend your knees with your feet flat on the bed and put your hands or even a pillow over the wound. If yours was a vaginal hysterectomy, put your hand firmly over the pad between your legs. Breathe deeply and cough out. However undignified you think it is, spit out the resulting spittle into a handkerchief.

The need to move around

Your throat could feel sore and your neck and shoulder muscles stiff. This is because during your operation the anaesthetist would have tipped your head backwards to allow a breathing tube to pass down your windpipe. The 'pull' on your muscles might leave you feeling a bit bruised. You could feel tired and find yourself sleeping twice as much as usual in the 24 hours after the operation. You may be surprised to find the nurses urging you out of bed as early as the first day, and almost certainly on the day after. Since you are supposed to be 'convalescing' or recovering, isn't this a bit brutal? Well, it isn't necessary for you to be flat on your back to rest. And the less movement you make, the greater the danger of your developing a post-operative thrombosis. This is when you get a blood clot in the veins in your legs. Sometimes, a clot travels through to your lungs, causing a pulmonary embolism, which is very dangerous. Even a healthy person who stays bedridden for a week has a one in seven chance of developing a clot in a leg vein. Surgery and a general anaesthetic increase the risk. But movement gets your blood flowing, which is why you will be chased out of bed as soon as possible and encouraged to walk around the ward.

The stitches will probably make it difficult for you to straighten up, forcing you to hobble around bowed over. As you heal, remind yourself to stretch upright and walk tall. If you have to stay in bed, you may be given drugs to thin your blood and prevent it from clotting. You will also be encouraged to exercise your legs. Wriggling your feet around and flexing the calf muscles regularly during the day will be as good as walking. It is important to do this. A pulmonary embolism *can* kill you, so these gentle exercises could save your life by preventing such a blood clot (see Appendix on p. 91). If you feel any pain or aching in your legs, find your ankles swelling, feel a pain in your chest especially when you breathe, are short of breath or have a dry cough, *tell the nurse immediately*.

There is a knack to getting out of bed in the early days, without straining those tender stomach muscles. Slide your feet up towards your buttocks, bending your knees. Then roll on to your side, keeping your knees bent, and push yourself into a sitting position with one or both hands while allowing your legs to swing down to the floor (see Appendix on p. 92). Walking around and chatting to your fellow patients will be a great help with the other aspect of your health, your emotions and feelings.

Post-operation blues

Two or three days after surgery, you may well get an attack of misery. There are several very good reasons for this. Surgery knocks you out, both physically and emotionally. A backlash of tears and tremors can hit anyone after any operation. Stress can affect the hormones or chemical messengers in your body, and these can trigger off feelings of fear and depression. If you have had your ovaries removed, your body will be adjusting to this loss. Menopausal symptoms can begin immediately, or in the fortnight following surgery. Even if your surgeon inserted an HRT implant in you during the operation or if you have been started on the tablets or patches, your body will still be adjusting. You may well be asked to wait and see if symptoms do occur. If they do you will be given therapy before leaving hospital or on your check-up visit. You can ask for pills to help you over this period. However, you may find it much better to have a heart-to-heart talk with the sister or a favourite nurse, or one of your fellow sufferers. Sharing your feelings and finding you are all roughly in the same boat does help. You may seesaw between feeling really good at finally getting rid of whatever problem led you to need a hysterectomy, and deep blues. Whatever your state of mind, it's normal, natural and part of the situation. So don't think you're going mad.

You might be puzzled and alarmed that neither the doctor nor the nurses actually say to you, 'The operation was a success.' If nothing particular is said, do not assume this means they aren't pleased or that something went wrong. However central the operation was to you and your life, it was a routine and common event to the medical staff. They expected it to go well!

Wind

A day or so after the operation, you may be allowed solid food. Unfortunately, since your gut is still likely to be less active than usual, you may develop wind. This sounds trivial – until it happens to you. Colicky pains can strike in your stomach and stab up through your body to your collar bone. When you are finally able to open your bowels or pass wind, the pains will go away. Till then, you may need pain relief. Some doctors and nurses will prescribe laxatives, suppositories or enemas to help.

Removing stitches

Five or six days after the operation, if you have an abdominal scar your stitches will be removed. Some doctors use plastic or metal clips instead of stitches. Whichever have been used, taking them out is an easy task. It's usually more scary and uncomfortable than painful. The stitches inside your body and in your vagina will be made of a dissolving thread and will take care of themselves. After the wound has been examined, you will get the all-clear to enjoy a relaxing soak in the bath. Up to now, you will only have been able to body wash or splash gently in a shallow tub.

Pain

You can't expect to go through what really, after all, is a major operation without experiencing some pain. However, the chances are that the anticipation may be worse than the actuality. We are all cowards at heart and it's perfectly normal not to want to be hurt. But the after-effects of a modern operation can be surprisingly light. Also, present-day pain relief is extremely effective. But you can't expect your doctors and nurses to read your mind and to know when and how much to help you unless you tell them how you are feeling. The good old British stiff upper lip is a real drawback. There's a second good reason to say if you're hurting. Quite apart from the discomfort it causes, the stress and trauma of pain is believed now to slow down the healing process. So the less pain you have to experience, the quicker you are going to get better. If you are hurting, don't just moan to your fellow patients or your family but say something to the staff. There is a wide range of treatment now, and if one thing doesn't work another may.

Exercises

Soon after your operation, a nurse or physiotherapist will show you a series of exercises (see Appendix on pp. 93–5). These are designed to strengthen the muscles bruised, stretched or cut during surgery. They may be tiring or even painful, but follow the instructions. They will include exercises to strengthen the muscles in your pelvic floor and belly. Neglect them, and you may find you suffer from backache and difficulty in holding your water. Your tummy will also sag, which it need not if you do these few stretches every day you are in hospital and during your convalescence. If at any time during this period you are in pain or discomfort, do not hesitate to ask a nurse for help. If you feel that your distress is not being taken seriously, do not give up but insist on seeing someone higher up. There is really no reason for you to suffer in silence.

Your family

It is important that during your stay you allow yourself to be looked after and not to worry about how your family is managing without you. Encourage them to visit you as often as you enjoy their visits, and do not be drawn into complaints or arguments about how everything has gone to rack and ruin without you. You might like to ask them to cheer you up with more than their presence, too. Hospital food has improved in many districts, but some still leaves a lot to be desired. If, when your appetite returns, you find yourself longing for a special treat, check with the sister to make sure it will do no harm, and place your order. Many a hospital patient has had their day 'made' by the arrival of a kind friend with a hamburger, steak sandwich or a tub of prawn cocktail. Chocolates and fruit are all very well, but something more substantial may be to your liking. Something alcoholic to share with your fellow patients when you're having your evening meal could be particularly welcome – but with this be especially careful. Ask the sister first, in case you or any of the others are on a treatment that does not go with alcohol.

Leaving hospital

About a week after the operation, you will be ready to go home. The surgeon or a member of the 'firm' will give instructions that you are ready and the sister or charge nurse will make arrangements with you. If you are alone at home or your family would be unable to look after you properly for the first two weeks, you could ask about the care that could be available. You might be able to get some home help. In some areas, you might be sent to a convalescence home, possibly in a country or seaside town. It would be free on the NHS or paid for by a union if you belong to one. This could offer a pleasant halfway house between the care of hospital and ordinary life.

In the bustle of leaving hospital, do not forget to get from the sister or the charge nurse:

- any medicines you need;
- your follow-up appointment to see the hospital doctor again in six to eight weeks' time;
- instructions on the exercises and the work you should and should not be doing for the next six to eight weeks;
- a signed National Insurance certificate, if you need it.

If you are going to a convalescence home or you have no transport, an ambulance or car will be arranged to collect you. Otherwise, you can now fix up for someone in your family or a friend to pick up your bags and take you home.

8
Going Home

I must admit I was spoiled rotten when I went home. The whole family ran round acting as if I was an invalid, and couldn't do enough for me. Very nice for a few days – but then I got bored. By this time, I was feeling fine, and they were still insisting I was ill. I put on a stone in weight with all the treats, and it took a lecture from our doctor to get them to allow me to do anything around the house. I know a lot of women have worse problems with bone-idle husbands and kids who won't help, but my lot really killed me with kindness.

Penny C

For most people, the first two weeks out of hospital are a time when special care is needed. The hospital would not send you home if they thought you needed *medical* care. But you will still need care of a sort. The physical after-effects of the operation will have left you weak and you are likely to tire easily. The operation cut, whether through the stomach or your vaginal wall, will make any physical work painful. Although the outer wound will have healed, the internal stitches will take five or six weeks to dissolve. Putting your stomach muscles under strain now won't burst these stitches. But you could pull uncomfortably against bruised and tender tissue, and may damage it. Emotionally, you may also feel rocky. Quite apart from any uneasiness you might have over the removal of your womb, your confidence will be shaken when you discover how little you can do at first. You will need to build up both your body and your self-confidence. You can be back to normal in three months or less. But you and your family and friends will have to understand what is going on and why, and agree to various compromises for this to be possible. The trick is to walk a fairly narrow line between your doing too much and too little.

There can be great temptations to rush through getting better as soon as you get home. If the house is in a mess, you might want to roll up your sleeves and get down to a spring-clean. Your family may be so relieved that you are home, safe, that they try to wipe out the memory of your illness by acting as if it didn't happen. Any sign on your part of tiredness, pain or irritation at their attitude may be met with annoyance. Their bad temper would probably be a screen for fears that you are still ill.

Alternatively, you could find yourself pampered beyond reason and treated as if you were still ill and in need of total care. Neither of these extreme attitudes would help you recover quickly. On your first evening home, you may find it a good idea to get all the family together and explain the 'plan of campaign'. Even small children will understand and want to help Mum or Granny when they are told, 'I can't do such and such yet but I will be able to in three weeks. Until then, you must help me slowly build up my strength.'

The first two weeks

For the first couple of days, you may want to stay close to home, if not actually indoors. Walking more than a few yards could leave you unsteady, so setting out for a long walk might be a mistake. Walking steadily round the house and then outside, in a garden, to the front gate or down the corridor outside a flat, will enable you to judge how far you can go. By the third day, you should be able to make a ten-minute or so walk a part of your daily routine. For the next six weeks, you should build this exercise up by five minutes a week. Just as when you were in hospital, walking is essential to stop blood clots forming in your legs, and to get you fit again.

For the first two weeks, however, this is about your limit. You may tire easily and could find an afternoon and even a mid-morning nap essential. Allow yourself this treat and don't feel lazy or selfish about it. Continue having a nap until you find even strong exercise leaves you able to go through a whole day without needing a rest. This will probably be after about four to six weeks of convalescence. You should not stand still for more than a few minutes, so cooking a family meal is out of the question. Get other people to cook or prepare meals. Keep yourself well supplied with things to read or watch during this time. You will have plenty of time for listening to the radio, watching television and reading books and magazines. Ask your family to ransack the library for you, and if you have a video, now is the chance for you to catch up on films the rest of the family don't like! Make a point, also, of reminding your friends and family that visits would be more appreciated *now*. This is when you need them, when you might be alone in the house all day, rather than in hospital, when you had plenty of company. Many people forget this obvious truth!

You will need to alternate sitting comfortably with short, careful walks. You can certainly take yourself off to the kitchen every now and then to make a cup of tea. However, rather than lifting the kettle, ferry water to it in cups, and when it boils, *tip* the contents into a jug or teapot, rather than lifting. You will have been told in hospital not to lift 'heavy' weights. How heavy is 'heavy'? The point to watch is whether the lifting brings your stomach as well as your arm muscles into action. Normally, tensing them would be automatic and unnoticed by you. With stitches in, you would soon feel the strain. The way you lift an object will be as important as its actual weight. Lifting a bag of sugar at arm's length will have the same effect as three times that weight close to your body. For the first two weeks, then, move nothing heavier than that kettle. Leave ironing and vacuuming for four to six weeks, lifting bags of shopping for at least six to eight weeks, and boxes and furniture for three months. When you do pick something up at last, do it properly. Hold your tummy in and, while keeping your feet slightly apart, bend at the knees. Take hold of the object and, keeping it close to your body, lift it by straightening your knees. In effect, you are trying to 'duck under' the weight, as a weightlifter does when he gets the bar above his waist level. This way, you take the strain off the stomach muscles.

How to lift a weight correctly

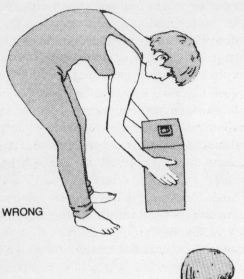

WRONG

RIGHT

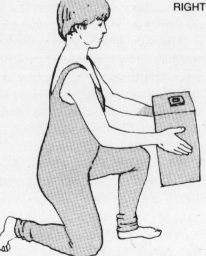

If you think that it will be impossible to keep to this total ban on lifting and standing for the first two weeks at home, either because you have no one to look after you or because other people will insist on you looking after them, then for your health's sake you *must* consider other options. Either accept the need to spend two weeks in a convalescence home or make sure the sister calls in the hospital social worker so that she can arrange for a home help. Your local social services department will send somebody, free, to clean up and prepare meals until you are able to do so yourself in perfect safety. You could, in fact, arrange this yourself with the social services department (the number will be in your local phone book) before you go into hospital.

The next two months

After the first two weeks, you will be able to increase your movement. You can do some light dusting, or the washing up, or cook a *quick* meal – as long as someone else carries pans of water or anything else that you feel 'pulls' on those muscles. Keep a stool or chair handy and sit down or prop your backside on it every now and then. Send someone else for the shopping or, if you would actually enjoy pottering around the local supermarket, take along a 'bag carrier'. That is, a human one, *not* a shopping trolley, since pulling one of these can be as much hard work as carrying your bags. Even young children can be surprisingly helpful if given trust and responsibility. So do not be afraid of recruiting 'child labour'!

After four weeks you can see if ironing and vacuuming is possible. Your body will be the best judge, and if your stomach 'twinges', take it easy. If you ache the following day, that is the signal to cut back on your timetable by a few days. As long as you can continue the gentle, pelvic-strengthening exercises the hospital will have shown you and increase your daily walks, you will find you regain your strength as the days pass. If you have a pleasant and not too crowded swimming pool nearby, you might like to consider using it. Swimming is the very best exercise

71

available, since it cushions your body at the same time as allowing you to stretch yourself. Visit as often as is comfortable, but keep in the shallow end just in case you overestimate your strength. By adding a width or two to your swim each time, you will soon build up those bruised muscles. But leave diving or jumping in until after your hospital follow-up visit.

An important aspect of your return to full health is your diet. It can be very tempting to give in to the relief of having come through the operation and illness and celebrate with edible treats. What better excuse for cream cakes or special chocolates? The problem is that, with your limited movement, this is how hysterectomy patients put on weight. *Not* as an inevitable result of the operation, but as a result of the treats afterwards! Being forced to take it easy can also have an effect on your bowels, making you constipated. The answer is to ensure that you get plenty of fresh fruit and vegetables. A fruit salad with yoghurt can be just as special and far better for you than fattening chocolates. To further make your bowels regular and help get your body trim, include wholewheat bread or pasta on that shopping list. Protein and calcium will also be a help, so ask for red meat, and especially iron-containing foods such as liver, fish and chicken, cheese and milk. To flush out your bladder and remove any last traces of an infection, drink plenty of liquids, particularly fresh fruit juices.

By the end of the sixth week at home, you should be moving around as normal, although you will find standing on your feet for any length of time is still tiring, and you will not yet be able to lift heavy objects. Although you could probably drive a car as soon as three to four weeks after the operation, it is a good idea to leave this until five to six weeks after your return home. Your concentration and co-ordination might have returned to normal before this, but resist the temptation. The danger is that if you have to stamp on the brake during an emergency stop, you could give yourself an extremely painful jolt in the belly.

It is quite likely that you will continue to have a discharge from the vagina during your first few weeks at home. This could be reddish-brown or yellowish in colour. If it does become stained with bright red blood or smells offensive, contact your doctor *at once*. Remember to use pads. A tampon would encourage infections.

Menopausal symptoms

If you had not yet been through the menopause and your ovaries were removed, you may well begin to have menopausal symptoms during your recovery. Even if you have been started on hormone replacement therapy (HRT), your body may take time to get used to the change and the dosage may need adjusting. Indeed, even if your ovaries were left intact, some women *do* experience menopausal symptoms either now or months after the operation. Although it is the ovaries that produce the majority of hormones to affect the whole of your body, it does appear that there could be a 'feedback' between uterus and ovary. Remove the uterus, and the ovaries respond. If you experience any of these symptoms, make a note and report them to your doctor on your follow-up visit:

- hot flushes, when your face and neck blushes and you feel a wave of heat;
- sweating, especially at night;
- palpitations, when your heart suddenly speeds up;
- difficulty in sleeping;
- depression;
- unexpected headaches;
- feelings of fear;
- difficulties in concentrating or remembering;
- unexplained loss of temper;
- unexplained tiredness;
- 'formication' – a feeling as if ants are crawling under your skin;
- a need to pass water too often;
- dryness in the vagina.

As many as seven out of ten women do experience a bout of depression after hysterectomy, and we shall discuss the emotional reasons for this in more detail in the next chapter. But, in some cases, the depression has a *physical* rather than an emotional root and would be helped by hormone replacement therapy. The loss of oestrogen from your system can have far-reaching and damaging effects. Even the natural menopause seems to be rather a bad joke at the expense of women. You can suffer uncomfortable symptoms of hot flushes. You may also find your vagina becomes dry and tender so lovemaking becomes painful or impossible. This can be upsetting in the extreme. Also, the loss of oestrogen causes bones to give up calcium. After the ovaries stop working, women lose as much as 1 per cent of the calcium in their bones each year. By the age of 70, a quarter of your bones could have leached away. Hardly surprising that old ladies are prone to hip fractures. The bones are so friable that they snap under the weight of the body. However, if oestrogen is given soon after the operation, even if treatment stops after a few years, it has a protective effect. It is also worth noting that a calcium-high diet and plenty of physical activity such as running or weight training has a bone-loading effect. This can protect against bone loss.

Few doctors now argue against the need for HRT when the ovaries have been removed. But many will argue that if yours are still intact any menopausal symptoms you report are psychological. By keeping a log and being ruthlessly honest with yourself, you can work out whether or not this may be true. If you are certain that your symptoms are physical in origin, do not allow yourself to be fobbed off, but persist until some doctor agrees to help you. If your doctor insists that there are medical reasons for oestrogen therapy being unsuitable for you, there is a range of treatments you can try to treat each symptom.

The first check-up

About six weeks after you have left hospital you will be asked to return for a check-up. You will see a member of the 'firm' that did your operation. Do not be surprised if this turns out to be a doctor you have not seen before. 'Junior' doctors can shift around with bewildering speed. Your hospital notes and access to the rest of the 'firm' will give him or her all the information needed to treat you properly. If your operation was through the abdomen, the doctor will look to make sure it has healed, without scar tissue building up. You will also be given an internal examination, to check that the wound at the top of the vaginal 'vault' where your cervix used to be has healed properly. Sometimes, tissue in the vagina builds up into 'granulated' tissue. This is a form of scar tissue. If so, the doctor may touch it with silver nitrate or another caustic solution, to burn it off, but you will not feel any pain at all. You might have to return a few times for the doctors to be sure that the granulations have gone. Very occasionally, the first you and your doctor know about them is when you start to bleed after making love, which can be a bit alarming.

Having checked you over, the doctor will give you the all-clear to go back to a normal life. You will usually be able to make love after this visit, and will be told when you can go back to work if you are employed outside the home. This will usually be eight to twelve weeks after leaving hospital. If you have to travel any distance by crowded public transport, you might like to arrange with your employer for you to travel outside rush hours for the first few weeks, so you can be sure of getting a seat. If they have not already, the doctors might now put you on HRT if they think it necessary. You could be given tablets or patches or have a tiny pellet inserted under the fatty layer on your stomach or backside. This would be done under local anaesthetic and take just a few minutes. You would be asked to return to your hospital or your own doctor for new prescriptions or implants every four to six months.

If you have *any* questions about your physical or emotional feelings, *ask the doctor*. He or she is paid by your taxes to look after you and give you a service. It's your body, and you both need and deserve the answers you want. If the hospital doctor really makes it impossible for you to get the answers you want, go and see your own general practitioner with your questions.

As well as making sure you know which type of hysterectomy you had, make sure you find out whether or not you need to continue having smear tests. Since your cervix has almost certainly been removed, these are rarely necessary. But if you had cancer or the doctor thinks you have reason for being a high cancer risk in the future, you may be asked to continue to have high vaginal smears. For these, a few cells would be collected from the top of the vaginal vault and these would be tested, just as with an ordinary Pap or smear test.

Recovering

It is not unusual to have a pot belly for some months after the operation. A haematoma – a bruise or a collection of blood in the tissue – could give you a lump under the wound, too. Both would take time to melt away as your body heals itself. As long as you do take sensible exercise and do watch your diet, there is no reason for your stomach to stay in this state, however. Ignore the myths that tell you it always takes six months to a year for a hysterectomy patient to recover. Unless you are in a particularly frail state or are unlucky, you should be recovered long before that. Obviously, there are cases when medical complications make recovery slow. But, in the main, how quickly you get well is in your hands. For the few months of your convalescence, you must put yourself first – often a very difficult task for a wife and mother used to looking after her family. If you can do this, giving yourself the proper mix of rest, exercise and good food, you will be fully fit by the third or fourth month after your operation.

9

How the Operation May Affect You

I felt absolutely hollow. I felt like a grapefruit which had been
cut open and had all the juice, all the flesh, all the goodness
scooped out. The first time we made love after the operation I
felt nothing. And I'll never forget the look of shock on John's
face as he entered me. After, he just kept muttering something
about it not being there any more. We couldn't make love
again for months.

Jenny B

The better prepared you are for your operation, the less likely you
are to be miserable afterwards. But even if you felt in control, you
may find yourself knocked sideways days, weeks or even months
later by a storm of confused emotions. You may feel grief, at the
loss of an important part of yourself or a chapter in your life. You
may experience anger that this had to happen to you. You may
feel as if your body has been trespassed upon and abused, and
your sexual attraction taken from you. Having been 'made
redundant' from one part of being a wife and mother – the job of
bearing children – you may find yourself doubting your ability to
do others. Can I really run a house as well as I did? Can I really
cook a meal as well as I did? Can I really be pleasing in bed, as I
once was?

Your family may contribute to these fears without realizing or
meaning to. They might be unhelpful to you and not understand
the need for a period of recovery. They all may act as if nothing
has happened, and assume that you are back to full health as soon
as you come out of hospital. They may complain about things
that have not been done and leave you feeling incompetent and
stupid. The only way they admit that you have been ill might be
to accuse you of being changed by the operation, as old standards
slide in the first few months. In such an atmosphere, it is hardly
surprising that the myths of 'You'll never be the same', 'You're
no good, you're less of a woman' become true, simply because

77

we believe it. You may become convinced that you are less capable and lovable, and so find it difficult to fight back and be either.

Sadly, the loving and caring family can have the same effect! If everyone rushes around, insisting that you are too frail to do anything, the chance to get back slowly into routines becomes harder. The first time you try anything – cooking, shopping, driving – and make a botch of it, you give yourself and your loving helpers another reason to insist you are not yet up to handling real life again. Worst of all, a gentle caring partner who 'spares you' his sexual attention at this time can leave you convinced that, as you feared, you are no longer sexually attractive.

Taking stock of your life

You may need to use the time during your convalescence to take stock of your life. If you recognize that your life is becoming stressed and pressures are beginning to tell, now is your opportunity to learn how to cope. You may have to reorganize your routines to give you times to relax. You may need to insist that your family step back so that you, rather than they, can come first in your priorities every now and again. You may need to make a sport or some form of exercise a part of your life. The very best way to burn off anger, relax tension and revitalize yourself is to spend half an hour jogging, swimming, walking or keeping fit.

You may need to get back into the habit of talking to your family and friends. If you can *explain* how you feel and why, you might be surprised at the results. Many people are awkward and embarrassed if they cannot understand what you are going through. Their embarrassment may increase briefly if you were to break the normal social rules of keeping a stiff upper lip and suffering in silence! But, very quickly, you would find that most of their apparent indifference to your plight was purely lack of information.

Sexual problems

Top of the list in any talk you have with your partner will be your love life. You may need to share how you view yourself and each other. After all, if both of you have always seen the main point of marriage as having children, where does your hysterectomy leave you now? You may need to take a good look at your marriage, to reassure yourself. Very few husbands really do see their wives as merely a housekeeper and a womb on legs. Friendship, companionship and loving, comforting sex are actually far more important if you were to be honest about it. In spite of all the tall stories and boasts, the vast majority of mature men do not want a young bed partner. They would rather have your maturity and understanding and the experiences you have shared over the years. None of this is easy to talk about openly, and you may be grateful for the help, support and advice of others. Your family doctor could give you this. Some health centres and doctors' partnerships have trained counsellors on the staff to deal with such discussions. Or you can approach your local branch of Relate. If you are lucky enough to have a Hysterectomy Support Group near you, you could share your experience with women and couples who have had, or are still trying to resolve, your dilemmas.

Unfortunately, a hysterectomy can often become necessary at just that age when other events put pressure on you and on your marriage. Your self-esteem, and that of your partner, can already be stressed by what is happening at home and at work. There may be job crises, as younger people challenge your authority and you feel you have reached the limit of your potential. Your children may be growing up, and need you less. You may already fancy that middle or old age has meant sexual love is supposed to be less important – but resent that fact.

With all this in the background, the first time you and your partner make love after the operation can be tense. There may be all sorts of unspoken needs and challenges. Your partner may have his own fears about what has happened, and these could have profound effects on his behaviour. These were discussed more fully in an earlier chapter. Your overwhelming need will be to have it proved to you that your partner *does* still find you a sexually exciting woman. And, just as important, that the operation has not stopped you experiencing sexual pleasure. Some doctors are fond of quoting one gynaecologist's reassuring joke: 'Madam, I have removed the baby carriage, not the playpen!' This is all very well, as long as you have not convinced yourself that you have no right to a playpen if the baby carriage is not in use!

You will probably have been asked not to have sex until after your check-up visit – about six weeks after you leave hospital. The main reason for this ban is that the wound at the top of the vagina, where your cervix was removed, needs time to heal up. Just as poking and prying at a scab with your fingers may open a cut, so your partner's penis may rub off newly formed tissue. This does not mean you should not have any form of sexual contact. Both of you may want to show your affection for each other and your thankfulness that you are home and on the way to recovery. You can 'make love' without having full intercourse. In the early days, though, you may find it painful to have an orgasm. This is because your orgasm triggers a complex series of muscular contractions in your body, and you may cause bruised and torn tissue to flex. You *cannot* damage yourself by this. But, just as clenching an arm muscle that has been bruised will hurt, so will these contractions. The main danger is that, like aversion therapy, the pain may put you off repeating the experience in case it happens again. Instead of enjoying lovemaking, you may find yourself unable to relax and let go because you are holding yourself ready against a stab of agony. If you can continue doing the exercises recommended by the hospital, you will be able to test for yourself when you are ready. In these, you will have been flexing the muscles in your abdomen and around your vagina. When you can grip hard, without an aching sensation, you will know you are safe.

In trying to be reassuring and to stop you feeling that sex is no longer for you, your doctors and nurses may be quite dogmatic. They may insist that the removal of your uterus, cervix and ovaries can have no physical affect on your and your partner's ability to make love and gain full pleasure from the experience. If you happen to be one of the couples who do have difficulties, you may be too embarrassed to ask for help. Or the help that is offered may be the wrong sort. The fact is that a hysterectomy can alter both your mind and body. Denial will not change the situation. But knowing how and why this could happen will allow you to remedy it.

Your sexual desire can be damped by all the above anxieties. It can, however, also be depressed by menopausal symptoms if your ovaries have been removed or if they have reacted to the disappearance of your uterus. If your menopause happened some time ago, having to take a rest from sexual activity while you were in hospital and getting better will also have made some uncomfortable changes. These will be worse if the illness leading up to your operation made you unwilling or unable to have sex. After the menopause, lack of oestrogen will tend to dry up the walls of the vagina and make them less stretchable. Regular sexual activity encourages the vagina to continue to produce moisture and to stay elastic and comfortable. You can find yourself, however, in a vicious circle – sex is painful, so you avoid it, allowing your vagina to atrophy (as these changes are called) even further. Sex becomes more unpleasant the less you try. Whether or not your ovaries were working before the operation, after at least two months of no sex and their removal or trauma, you may well find a sexual approach by your partner does not make you feel sexy or moist. And even if you do feel aroused and ready for sex, your vagina may remain dry and uncooperative.

There is one circumstance where your partner may be able to feel a difference during sex after you have had a hysterectomy. This is when your operation was for large and numerous fibroids. During sexual excitement, the ligaments that hold up the womb tighten. They draw your womb up into the pelvic cavity so that your partner's thrusts will not be painful. A uterus made bulky with fibroids may stay in a low position. Since the fibroids would have grown over a period, you and your partner would not have noticed the fact that you make allowances for this in the way you make love. What is more, you and your partner may have become used to the sensation of tightness or fullness at the top of your vagina. Even though the space left by the uterus is filled instantly by intestine and other organs, in contrast to the bulky, full uterus, both of you may feel something is missing when your partner thrusts for the first time.

Even your orgasm can be affected. There used to be a belief that there were two types of orgasm, clitoral and vaginal. It was thought that clitoral orgasms were childish, and that in the process of maturing a woman shifted her sexual feelings from the clitoris to the vagina. This is now known to be untrue. All female orgasms occur when the clitoris is stimulated. This stimulation can be direct. The clitoris can be rubbed with a finger or react to pressure between your and your partner's bodies. Or it can be indirect, with the clitoral hood brushed to and fro against this organ by the movement of his penis in your vagina. This is transmitted through the muscles and tissue of your vulva. There is also now increasing evidence that, in spite of the cervix and the upper two-thirds of your vagina having few nerve endings, many women are stimulated by the sensation of their partner's penis butting against the cervix and uterus. Furthermore, during orgasm we know that not only the vagina but also the uterus and the ligaments that hold it in place tighten and spasm. If the womb and its supports are taken away, some of the muscular ripples that excite the clitoris to its explosion of pleasure are removed as well.

This is not to say that hysterectomy destroys sexual pleasure. It certainly need not. But if you were one of the people whose orgasm was in part a result of such movements, you may need to re-explore your body and re-educate its responses. You could do this by experimenting with sexual positions and more direct caresses to the clitoris itself. Many women find that orgasm after a hysterectomy is a sharper and more intense sensation. Your feelings can be localized on your clitoris, rather than diffused and spread out. For this reason, some women say the experience can be even more satisfying.

There is no point in pretending that your hysterectomy will

leave you untouched and exactly the same person as you were before. The mistake we make, however, is believing that 'different' has to mean 'worse', or even 'better'. You are a different person now from the one you were as a teenager. If you are partnered or a mother, you are different from the person you were as a single woman or a non-parent. All experiences change you, and the trick is recognizing in advance that this will be so and taking steps to ensure you like the result. Using your convalescence to take control of your life, and to communicate with the people to whom you are close, can certainly make 'different' into 'better'.

10

Some Common Questions

Can I avoid having a hysterectomy?

There is evidence to show that your lifestyle has an important effect on your health. Being a non-smoker, a moderate drinker, eating fresh and healthy food and enjoying regular exercise may reduce your risk of much illness. Having regular check-ups and going to your doctor as soon as you suspect there is anything wrong could help you to avoid the need for a hysterectomy. There are quite a few conditions that can be detected and treated easily *before* they become dangerous. Cancer of the cervix, the most common cancer leading to hysterectomy, is the most obvious.

But what if your doctor suggests a hysterectomy and you don't want one? Your body belongs to you and you have every right to refuse any type of medical treatment, whatever the circumstances. Clearly, if you had cancer or a serious case of pelvic inflammatory disease, endometriosis or fibroids and your doctor advised you to have an operation, you would be unreasonable to refuse. But there are times when more conservative treatment could work. Some of the conditions that lead to hysterectomy would respond to drug treatment or surgery to remove the site of the problem alone. You and your doctor should certainly discuss trying alternative treatment before moving on to surgery.

Can I do anything before the operation to speed up my recovery afterwards?

Get fit and get your eating patterns sorted out. The more exercise you do before your op, the better you'll feel. You'll also then be in the habit of doing some fitness routines. When you're feeling better, you can return to them again. Go to a fitness class twice to three times a week. Or take a brisk walk, run or cycle most days. Look at what you eat. Cut out fat and extra sugar. Don't eat fried food and only have cakes, biscuits or puddings as special treats.

And eat at least five portions of fresh fruit, fruit juice, salad and vegetables each day.

Will I get depressed after a hysterectomy?

It used to be taken for granted that every woman having a hysterectomy would suffer depression. We now realize that this is not necessarily true. Any operation can be a shock to the system, both physically and emotionally. Your body can react some days after with rapid mood changes that are beyond your control. And being in a strange place, away from your family, and having just had your childbearing years brought forcefully to a close can make anyone weepy. But the higher figures for depression among hysterectomy patients probably occur more from lack of proper care and guidance than from the operation itself.

Recent studies suggest, however, that women who have had information and an opportunity to talk about the operation experience far fewer problems than hysterectomy patients once did, and no more than after any other type of surgery. The more you know, the more you talk about what is happening and the more you feel in control, the easier it will be to cope. Depression often happens when you have to bottle up a worry or a misery and cannot share it with anyone. Being able to cry openly and to make it clear when and why you feel upset, both in hospital and when you go home, will help you to get over these feelings quickly.

Will a hysterectomy make me fat?

The short answer is that a hysterectomy operation will not, in itself, make you put on weight. But, of course, some people do get fatter afterwards, and this is why this myth persists. Immediately after the operation, you may find your belly bulges out alarmingly. This is because the tissues around your incision will be swollen. If you have a haematoma – another word for a bruise – this will add to the lumpy appearance of your tummy. As you try solid food for the first time after the operation, your bowels may have difficulty in working and you may 'blow up' with wind. As you stagger round in the first days on your feet, you could look down on what to your horror appears to be a pregnant tummy! This is only temporary. It will go down in a few days, and the lump under the operation site will disappear over the next few months.

However, with having to rest at home you might get into the habit of eating more food than your body is using in energy. It is this that may well lead to your putting on weight. If you can keep an eye on your diet and make some sort of exercise a part of your routine, you will find that fat and hysterectomy do not have to go together.

Does a hysterectomy mean my sex life is over?

We have sex for many reasons, not just to make babies. We also 'make love' – showing our affection and desire and reaffirming our companionship. Just because pregnancy is no longer a possibility does not mean that these other reasons lose their significance. Unfortunately, in this society we do tend to believe the ridiculous myth that only 'the young and the beautiful' have sex. So we think that no longer being able to become pregnant means you are old – and old sex is dirty and undignified. What nonsense! Whatever your age and your physical condition, sexual expression is rightfully yours.

Having your womb removed will not 'sew up' your vagina or sex passage. The cervix or neck of the womb which juts out into the top of the passage will be gone, but neither you nor your partner are likely to feel the slightest difference when you have sex. Only in very rare cases does the surgeon have to shorten the vagina by removing the top third. Even then, lovemaking can be unaffected. Sex doesn't have to be penetrative to be satisfying.

Will hysterectomy make me less of a woman?

It is not your womb that makes you female. Your femininity is locked into every cell in your body. You were female before you could have children and will still be so after this ability is gone. It is true that a small part of our sexual desires depends on the hormones or chemical messengers that are secreted by the ovaries. If these are removed during a hysterectomy, some women do find their sexual feelings become less, as they can after natural menopause. But more women find their sex drive is unaffected by this event. It can even be increased as unplanned or unwanted pregnancies become impossible.

Although hormones play a part, desire is more an emotional than a physical response. Some women do not like sex without the possibility of pregnancy. If you see being a mother as the most important part of your existence, you may feel that having your womb removed mutilates you. These are not unusual feelings. But they are more a reflection of our society's rather unfair attitude to women than a true estimate of your worth. An operation to remove any part of your body leaves you as human and as feminine as before. It is your attitude and the attitudes of those around you, not the surgeon's knife, that may change things. Which means that refusing to accept these foolish and harmful beliefs robs them of their ability to harm you.

Will I take ages to get over having a hysterectomy?

Everyone will tell you about a friend, or a friend of a friend, who took months or even years to recover from their operation. You can easily become convinced that a hysterectomy condemns you to the life of an invalid. This is just not true. Obviously, if your operation is made necessary by a long and exhausting illness, or if you need drug therapy or radiotherapy to complete the cure, you may take some time to regain your full health. But it will be the illness and the operation as an added strain that puts you in this situation. The older you are, the slower you will be to shrug off both major surgery and the wasting effects of bed-rest. But even 'senior citizens' can bounce back from this operation.

If you go into the operating theatre in average health, for an average hysterectomy, and follow sensible advice about rest, diet and exercise, you should be back to normal in three to four months.

Will a hysterectomy make me masculine?

The fear that a hysterectomy makes you manly could come from the fact that women lacking in oestrogen sometimes find facial hair becomes longer and thicker. In unusual cases, it can actually resemble a sparse moustache or beard. However, this happens very, very rarely. The use of hormone replacement therapy (HRT), to replace lost oestrogen in women who have lost functioning ovaries, means that it is most unlikely to happen to you. Having lost your womb, you are still *genetically* a woman and nothing will change that fact!

Will a hysterectomy age me prematurely?

The end of childbearing has always been associated with old age. There is some truth in this myth. When your ovaries are not at work secreting oestrogen into your body, various changes happen. As well as the uncomfortable symptoms of the menopause – hot flushes and night sweats, headaches, depression, anxiety and tiredness – you can find your skin becoming wrinkled and dull and your hair lacklustre and thin. Worst of all, your bones may become fragile and your arteries may harden and thicken. If your ovaries are removed before the natural menopause, all these changes could become noticeable and happen before you would expect them. However, none of this need occur as a result of hysterectomy. Your ovaries may well be left untouched and only your womb removed. If both ovaries do have to go, your doctor will prescribe treatment to replace all the oestrogen your ovaries are no longer able to give you. This is called hormone replacement therapy (HRT), and it should be available to any woman who needs it. If there are no medical reasons for you not to have HRT and your hospital or family doctor is unwilling to prescribe it, you may find there is a specialist clinic at a nearby hospital who will help. Your local family planning clinic may also be able to assist you.

Are there any advantages to having a hysterectomy?

There most certainly are! If you haven't had your menopause yet, you'd still be having to cope with periods and birth control. After a hysterectomy, you will never have to worry about periods again. Nor will you have to bother about contraception. If the illness that led to your operation made you feel dragged down and tense and gave you cramps or pain, all this will go. You may find as you get better and recover fully that you feel more energetic and optimistic than you have for years. Having to take a rest might give you a chance to take stock of your life. You may be able to take a fresh look at your relationships with partner, family and friends and improve them. For all these reasons, many women find that their lives are better after the operation than they have been for some years.

Appendix: Exercises and Manoeuvres

If you have to stay in bed for more than a day after your operation, try these exercises to keep the blood in your legs moving:

Foot stretch

Keeping your legs straight, point your toes and then flex your foot towards you, ten times.

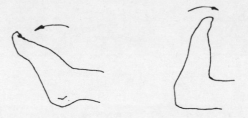

Foot circle

Keeping your legs straight, circle your feet round, ten times each way.

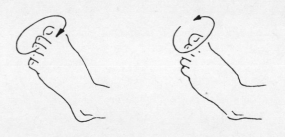

Getting out of bed

When you want to get out of bed, try this method to take the strain off your sore tummy:

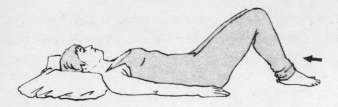

Slide your feet towards your body, so your knees are bent.

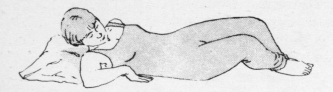

Roll on your side and begin to push yourself up on one arm, keeping your knees bent.

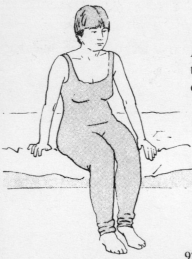

As you push up, allow your legs to swing down, so your feet are on the floor.

The hospital physiotherapist will probably show you these exercises to do, from the day after your operation.

Pelvic floor exercise

While lying down or sitting, pull in the muscles around your back passage, your vagina or sex passage, and your front passage. You will find you can do this as if you were trying to hold in your water or stop a bowel motion, or as you would 'pull in' as you felt menstrual blood leak out. Hold tightly and count to four, then release slowly. Repeat this five times. Try not to hold your breath as you do this exercise, and do it as often as possible. If you have always had good muscle tone (if you could stop yourself in the middle of passing water) then three times a day would be enough. Otherwise, every hour or two would be wise. This exercise helps you regain tone and control of the muscles in your pelvis. If you neglect them, you may find the muscles become slack and water can leak out when you laugh, sneeze or run.

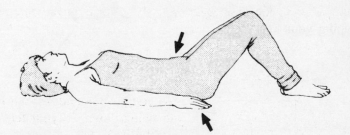

Pelvic tilt exercise

Lie on your back with a pillow under your head and your knees bent. Pull in your tummy, and by tilting your bottom slightly towards the ceiling, try to flatten your back against the floor or mattress. Without holding your breath, count to four and then relax. Repeat this five times. Done lying on your back, this exercise not only relieves backache but can clear wind. As you get better, if you do it while standing it will improve your posture.

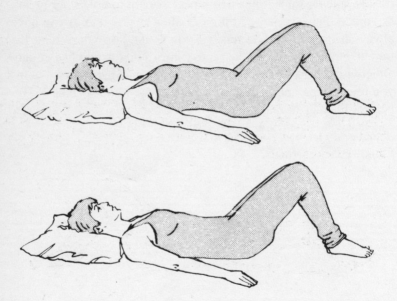

After your stitches have been removed, you will be asked to tone up your stomach muscles a bit more. You should do the following exercises at least three times a day.

Stomach muscle tightening

While lying on your back or standing, pull in and hold your stomach muscles. Count to four, then relax. Repeat five times.

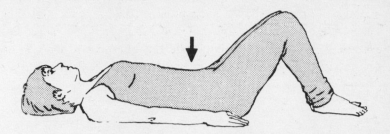

Stomach muscle strengthening

Lie on your back with your head on a pillow and your knees bent. Tuck your chin in, rest your hands on your thighs and lift your head up to look at your knees. Count to four and relax slowly. Do this five more times.

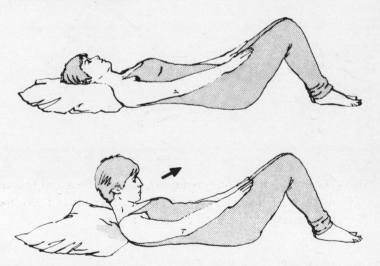

As you get better, add an extra repetition of exercises each day.

Useful Addresses and Information

Hysterectomy Support Network
c/o Women's Health
52 Featherstone Street
London EC1Y 8RT.
Tel: 020 7251 6580

These are self-help groups giving hysterectomy patients and partners the chance to share their experiences and views, and pool information and support.

The National Endometriosis Society
50 Westminster Palace Gardens
Artillery Row
London SW1P 1RL.
Tel: 020 7222 2776
www.endo.org.uk

A national helpline and self-help groups and information for endometriosis sufferers.

Women's Nutritional Advisory Service
PO Box 268, Lewes
East Sussex BN7 2QN.
Tel: 01273 487366
www.wnas.org.uk

An advice and information service, particularly concerned with diet. Booklets and information pack. Fees charged.

Relate

Herbert Gray College,
Little Church Street, Rugby
Warwickshire CV21 3AP.
Tel: 01788 573241
(All branch addresses are listed in local telephone directories.)
www.relate.org.uk

Offers fully trained counsellors to help you work through any relationship, emotional or sexual problems.

Family Planning Association

2–12 Pentonville Road
London N1 9FP.
Tel: 020 7837 5432
www.fpa.org.uk

The Association publishes leaflets and information sheets on many aspects of sexual health.

Index

ageing 89

biopsies, cone 24
bleeding 30; between periods 30; post-operative 59–60, 72–3
blood clots: elastic stockings 54; post-operative exercise 60–1, 68

calcium 74
cancer 19, 23–4, 31; cervical 24; endometrial 24–5; necessity of hysterectomy 85; ovarian 25
catheters 58–9
cervix 75–6; cancer of 24, 85
communication: information about hysterectomy 5; with partners 10–12
consent forms 52–4
contraceptive pills: correcting hormone imbalance 33; stopping 48

depression *see* emotions
dilatation and curettage (D & C) 23
doctors: and emotional reactions 3–4; first post-operative check-up 74–6; at

hospital 51–2; internal examination 20–2; relationship with 35–6
driving 72
dysmenorrhoea 30, 32

elastic stockings 54
emotions: deep reactions 1–4; factors influencing 5–6; general coping ability 6; long-term effects 77–8; nervousness about hospitals 47–8; post-op blues 61–2, 73–4, 86; recovering confidence 67
endometriosis 19, 25–6, 31; total hysterectomy 43
endometrium 17; ablation and resection 34–5; cancer of 24–5
exercise: long-term recovery 71–2, 78; pelvic strengthening 71, 93; post-operative 63–4, 91–5; pre-operative 48–9, 85–6; prevention of blood clots 60–1, 68

Fallopian tubes 15, 42–3
family 5; children's reaction 7–8; pre-operative